Overcoming Dyslexia
A Practical Handbook for the Classroom

Overcoming Dyslexia: A Practical Handbook for the Classroom

by Hilary Broomfield and Margaret Combley

Consultant in Dyslexia: Professor Margaret Snowling
University of York

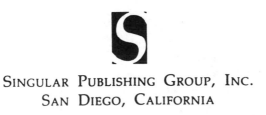

SINGULAR PUBLISHING GROUP, INC.
SAN DIEGO, CALIFORNIA

© 1997 Whurr Publishers Ltd

First Published 1997 by
Whurr Publishers Ltd
19b Compton Terrace, London N1 2UN, England

Published and Distributed in the
United States and Canada by
SINGULAR PUBLISHING GROUP, INC.
401 West A Street, Suite 325
San Diego, CA 92101, USA

British Library Cataloguing in Publication Data
A catalogue record for this book is available from the British Library.

ISBN 1-86156-008-7

Singular Number 1-56593-836-4

Drawings by Rosalind Combley

This book is printed on paper of high purity
and free from acid producing chemicals.
Printed and bound in the UK by Athenaeum Press Ltd,
Gateshead, Tyne & Wear

Contents

Part 2: Skills into Action

Part 3 The Step-by-Step Programme

Preface

This book has taken two years to write but has been fifteen years in the making. It is the result of the culmination of experience of two practising teachers in the field of language and literacy difficulties. Our complementary backgrounds in the areas of dyslexia, speech and language disorders have come together in this volume to produce something that we believe is new and exciting—a truly integrated, structured approach to overcoming literacy difficulties. The teaching programme has been developed through an interactive and evolving process, our ideas being refined through ongoing work with children and young people. We have drawn on these experiences and on case studies of our learners in presenting our approach.

Our aim has been to bring together the best of practice in the areas of multi-sensory teaching, whole language, and phonological awareness training, to produce a programme that integrates skills teaching into real reading and writing. Although intended as a teacher-friendly, 'hands on' approach, it is firmly rooted in recent research into the development of reading and writing, and into the causes of literacy difficulties. We have been particularly excited by two approaches. One is set out in Marilyn Jager Adams' (1990) book *Beginning to Read*. This classic work presents a view of reading that should resolve the debate on 'phonics versus real books' that has dogged generations of teachers. The second important approach is the work that connects literacy and language difficulties, and seeks common ground with communication therapists and speech scientists.

We hope that fellow practitioners in the areas of language and literacy will find much of use here. Our readership might include teachers, speech and language therapists, and educational psychologists. Our ideas have already formed part of in-service training courses for teachers and therapists, and other professionals providing in-service training to these groups might appreciate our approach. Our work alongside speech and language therapists over the years has resulted in a cross-over of knowledge, and we have assimilated techniques used by therapists into our own practice. The ideas for linking teaching skills into reading and writing contexts will appeal to teachers who are aiming to produce individual education programmes for learners with literacy difficulties.

Our approach has been used with learners with dyslexia, speech and language disorders, and with those experiencing more general learning difficulties of a mild to moderate nature. There are no age barriers—we have worked with young children just beginning school and with young people just about to leave. The techniques can be used by them all, as long as attention is paid to the interests and maturity of the learner, and care is taken in choosing age-appropriate materials.

We do not assume previous knowledge on behalf of the learner; our programme aims to assess individual knowledge, skills and weaknesses, and to build up a detailed profile, with practical ways forward for further learning. The key features apply to all ages: the importance of firm foundations in spoken language; the understanding of the nature and purpose of print; the building up of an awareness of the sounds within spoken language; and the development of automatic sound symbol links.

We owe much to the learners we have worked with along the way, and to the many hours of discussion we have had with fellow teachers, and speech and language therapists. We would like to give our particular thanks to the staff, parents and children at the Rowan School in Sheffield. We are forever indebted to them for their enthusiasm and commitment to the literacy learning process.

Part 1: Background

This first section establishes the research background for our teaching approach. It puts forward the view of literacy as a language learning process and looks at the specific language and literacy of the dyslexic learner. Case studies from the authors' own experience are used to inform the research. The importance of phonological awareness and the use of analogy in reading is stressed. A model of reading from Marilyn Jager Adams' book *Beginning to Read* is used to establish the need for an integrated approach to literacy. Some common approaches to the teaching of reading are discussed along with their implications for the dyslexic learner. More specialised approaches such as multisensory teaching, cued articulation and rebus symbols are described. From this wealth of research and tradition, there emerges the need for a teaching programme that integrates good practice from whole language approaches, multisensory teaching methods, and training in phonological awareness: a teaching programme that enables the learner to develop new skills, and to put these skills into action.

Chapter 1:
Language and Literacy

Literacy as a Language Process

From the very moment we are born we begin to develop language. We learn how to respond to and to interact with others, building relationships with them through our communication skills. We develop our thinking and understanding of the world through language and through our interactions with others. Through time, our civilised society has developed a further mode of communication, that of written language. Our society and culture is now built around the ability to interpret and use this. If for some reason we have difficulty in interpreting this written code, then we are denied full access to the culture that has developed around it.

For those of us who read and write fluently, it is difficult to imagine the pain (and for some, the shame) of being set apart in this way. Each day is filled with aspects of written language: reading a bus timetable, writing a shopping list, interpreting a bill, reading the local paper or the latest best-seller. Each day, fluent readers carry out these activities automatically, moving between spoken and written language with ease. The two modes of communication are inextricably linked. As teachers of young people with reading and writing difficulties, we need to understand these links if we are to help them crack the code.

Although based on spoken language, written language is not just spoken language written down. There are similarities but there are also essential differences making interpretation of the code complex. A look at some of these may help us as teachers to understand some of the difficulties our learners face, (see Table 1.1).

In order to become fluent at reading and writing, the learner needs experience, knowledge and competence in understanding and using spoken language, along with experience and knowledge of the world. This language and experience base is in turn supported by the learner's own physical, cognitive and memory skills. Many of our learners have difficulties in these areas even before they begin to try and crack the written code. If they are then mapping their new learning onto a faulty language base, it is no wonder that they struggle to make sense of it all. Understanding spoken language, language development and language difficulty is an essential part of the teacher's knowledge of how to approach such learners.

Table 1.1

Spoken language:	Written language:
is transient and sequenced in time: it can only be heard again if the speaker repeats it, or if it is recorded on tape.	is more permanent, occurs in space, and has directionality across the page. It can be scanned again to aid understanding.
is an arbitrary code that we use to represent our thoughts and ideas.	is a further code on top of this.
consists of 40 plus phonemes (speech sounds).	has graphemes—26 letters of the alphabet that singly or in combination represent these phonemes. One letter can represents different phonemes (e.g. c in cat, city).
is a continuous stream of sound patterns with unclear breaks between words.	has letters grouped together to represent words with clear spaces between them.
is sociable and interactive— meaning is bound to and supported by context. Meaning can be checked by participants.	tends to be more solitary—there is no shared context, and writer and reader are not usually able to negotiate meaning.
is aided by non-verbal clues such as gesture, intonation, facial expression, etc.	has punctuation, underlining and spelling to aid meaning, but with less effect.
tends to be informal, variable, easier to produce.	is more formal, standard, with its own literary style and conventions; tends to be harder to produce.

A Model of Language

Lahey's (1988) model of spoken language may help us get a clearer picture. The model refers to both the use and understanding of language and illustrates and explains the different dimensions involved. There are three main headings: form, content and use. Each area supports and interacts with the other two.

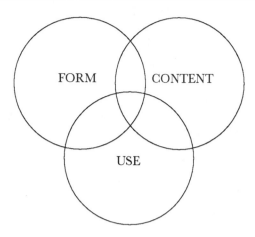

Figure 1.1 Lahey's model of spoken language

Form refers to the sounds, syllables, stresses, rhythm and intonation that we use when we speak (phonology). It also includes our arrangement of words and grammatical inflections within a sentence according to meaning (syntax and morphology).
Content is concerned with the ideas and meaning behind these sounds, words and structures (semantics).
Use refers to the way language changes in different situations and with varying conversational partners—how and why we speak (pragmatics).

Each time we speak, we simultaneously use the different dimensions of the model to articulate, produce, organize and express what we want to say and how we want to say it. The words we use and the way in which we say them will vary according to whom we are speaking, and to where we are. Lahey's model illustrates this successful communication by overlapping form, content and use. It is easy to see how written language could have a similar model to describe it. Through the use of such models teachers and researchers are moving towards a solid understanding of written language, and its relationship to spoken language.

Language Development

Young children learn the sound, structure and meaning of spoken language through their social interactions with adults. (Bruner, 1983; Vygotsky, 1978). Familiar routines such as bedtime, bathtime and mealtimes are full of language learning. Parents help their children to join in these activities and respond to their communication attempts, gradually increasing their expectations. The term 'scaffolding' has been used to describe this adult support. Just as scaffolding round a building provides a supportive framework to enable work to be carried out, so does an adult provide support and guidance to enable a young child to achieve at a higher level than when alone. The child, supported by an adult, is actively involved and responds to the familiar routines and language. The adult in turn responds to the language and actions of the child. The learning is truly collaborative and the child's experience and confidence in using language grows. More recent approaches to the teaching of reading have tried to emulate this (see Shared Reading, p 61).

Experience and confidence in using language are important, but not enough for the young reader or writer. They also need to be able to think and talk about aspects of language as if they are objects that can be manipulated or discussed. Metalinguistic skill (i.e. using language to talk about language) is crucial to classroom talk and literacy learning. It may develop as a consequence of learning to read (Donaldson, 1978) or before (Tunmer and Bower, 1984). The development may be intermingled (Garton and Pratt, 1989, Van Kleek, 1984), but teachers need to be aware of its importance in teaching programmes. Just think of how many times we ask children to talk about 'words', 'sounds' and 'letters' as we go about our teaching. Our learners need to understand these concepts if they are to make sense of this classroom talk. They need to develop such skills in order to understand how the written code is mapped onto spoken language. We should not assume that our learners already understand these terms.

Attention Skills

Attention skills are an important aspect of language and learning. Children making slow progress in literacy often exhibit attentional difficulties. These may be related to motivation, physical well-being, or emotional factors, but may also be developmental in nature, springing from an inability to integrate incoming information from different sensory channels. Those working with such children need to be aware of the difficulties and to ensure that work and expectations are set within the capabilities of the child's developmental level. Severe difficulty in this area, Attention Deficit/Hyperactivity Disorder (ADHD), is now recognized as a learning disability. Teachers of children with extreme difficulties in attention will need the guidance of an educational psychologist. Reynell (see Cooper, Moodley and Reynell 1978) outlined a developmental framework that is a useful guide in assessing attention and in developing our learning programmes.

First Stage (0 to 1 year)

This stage is characterized by extreme distractibility. The child's attention is sustained only fleetingly.

Second Stage (1 to 2 years)

The child is able to focus on self-chosen tasks in a single channelled way, but is unable to accept adult involvement without losing concentration.

Third Stage (2 to 3 years)

The child may be able to accept such involvement, but is unable to listen and carry out an activity at the same time; adult help is needed if the child is to stop and focus on instruction.

Fourth Stage (3 to 4 years)

Adult help is no longer needed in stopping an activity in order to focus on an instruction, although the child still needs to stop when listening.

Fifth Stage (4 to 5 years)

Concentration span is still short, but the child is able to listen to an instruction related to a task without interrupting the activity. The child can work in a group.

Sixth Stage (5 to 6 years)

Attention is well established, integrated and sustained.

Such a framework can help teachers recognize children with a specific difficulty in attending to and integrating information. We need to acknowledge that there are many children starting school who are still unable to attend to instruction and work on a task simultaneously, or who are so distracted by extraneous noise or visual activity that concentration on the teacher or the task becomes impossible. For such children the teaching and learning environment, and the language of instruction, may need to be modified. The teacher cannot assume or expect a mature level of attention control. For some children with extreme difficulties it may be necessary to work directly in this area (see Cooke and Williams, 1985) before embarking on direct teaching of literacy skills.

Spoken Language Difficulties

Lahey's model of spoken language can also be used to illustrate a speech or language problem. One or more of the circles may become separated from the others. Children may experience, for example, difficulty with the form of language in articulating speech sounds, organizing words into sentences, or in using the correct tense. Problems with language content and use could be illustrated in a similar way. Imagine, for example, not being able to express ideas fluently because you keep forgetting the words you want to use; imagine having no understanding of the need to choose appropriate vocabulary and tone when talking to a stranger instead of a close friend.

Think how such difficulties might affect written language, perhaps in spelling or decoding a word, in predicting and using correct vocabulary, or in the construction and interpretation of a meaningful piece of prose. The literature points to a strong correlation between difficulties in spoken language and difficulties in learning to read and write. (Bryant and Bradley, 1985; Goswami and Bryant, 1990; Snowling, 1987; Stackhouse, 1989, 1990; Stackhouse and Wells, 1992).

Speech and language difficulties are not always apparent at a surface level, but there may be a past history of such problems. Early difficulties with speech sounds, syntax or narrative do not disappear, but may be transferred directly to those same areas of written language (Maxwell and Wallach, 1984). Research suggests that if a child had difficulty in analysing speech sounds at the age of 6, there are likely to be continuing problems with reading and spelling three years later, even though the difficulty with sounds in the child's own speech is no longer apparent (Fox and Routh, 1983)

If there is a 'faulty' base of poor speech and language competence, perhaps combined with poor metalinguistic skills, there may be difficulties in literacy learning as the child tries to map the written code onto the spoken one. Particular difficulties seem to occur as the child tries to learn phonic skills. If there are significant difficulties with spoken communication then the advice of a communication therapist should be sought.

Readers will find many useful practical ideas in Cooke and Williams' (1985) *Working With Children's Language Disorders*. Lees and Urwin (1991) explain the background to such disorders, and give illustrative case studies and ideas for learners from pre-school to teenage in *Children With Language Disorders*.

The language processes involved in fluent reading and writing are complex. In trying to understand them we can begin to see where the difficulties lie and how we can help.

A Model of Reading

In her book *Beginning to Read* Adams (1990) puts forward a useful model of the reading process (see fig 1.2) that helps us understand the different routes and strategies that successful readers use as they encounter print. Adams refers to different 'processors' that interact with each other, further refining how each one responds. This model links with the form, content and use of Lahey's model of spoken language.

The *orthographic processor* is concerned with a reader's visual response to print, to the letters, letter sequences, and whole words.

The *phonological processor* responds to the sounds involved as we read both silently and aloud. It is not only concerned with word attack, as subvocalization aids both memory and comprehension. Within this processor we have auditory 'images' of phonemes, syllables, onsets and rime (see p.26-27.).

The reader's *meaning processor* gives meaning to individual words and morphemes (e.g. suffixes, prefixes and wordroots).

The *context processor* takes a broader view, refining this initial meaning according to the situation, helping us to respond to the text or the book as a whole.

Note that there are two-way links between the processors. Adams suggests that these links are important as each single processor constantly guides and facilitates the efforts of the others. Let us take an example of word reading ('roll') to help us through the model. As we look at the word 'roll' we respond to the visual shape of the word and the letter strings it contains (orthographic processor).

To help us respond more accurately, we can turn these visual images into sound through our knowledge of letter–sound correspondence and pronounce the

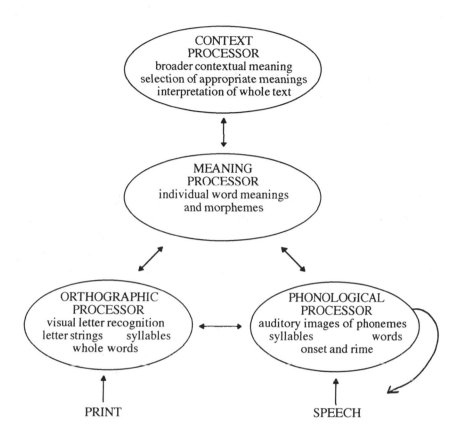

Figure 1.2 Adams' model of reading

This joint information may lead us to understand that the word is a verb that means turning over and over, rather than the part that an actor plays in a film (meaning processor).

However, if we are reading a chapter in a cookery book about making bread, the placement of the word in the sentence may make it clear that the word is a noun and not a verb. We only need the accompanying word 'granary' to confirm the real meaning as a small rounded loaf of bread! (context processor).

Of course the route to reading and understanding may vary. If we are reading a word we have read a hundred times before, then the visual recognition of the word and its meaning may happen almost instantly. Adams (1994) states that a skilled reader can read more than 300 words a minute. Unfamiliar words will take longer. Research suggests that the processing that takes place when skilled readers read happens so quickly that they are unaware of what has happened (Just and

Carpenter, 1987; Patterson and Coltheart, 1987). Although text is read from left to right, word by word, and *letter by letter*, the process is both automatic and effortless, and therefore unnoticed. Think of the many daily activities we carry out, such as walking, speaking, driving a car. We do not think about the individual skills and movements that make up these activities, we just do them. It is the same for the skilled reader. It is only when we are learning something new or doing something that we find difficult that we become more conscious of the processes that are involved.

Adams' model has guided us through the complexities of reading and has shown us that there is no single route to success. Each aspect of the process mutually informs and supports another. The routes we take to identifying words will depend on our ability to make use of the range of information available. This has to have implications for how we teach reading and how we might begin to help those experiencing difficulty. It confirms the view that skills, visual, phonic, or contextual, should not be taught in isolation. The teacher needs to adopt approaches that will encourage the learner to use the skills in an integrated and purposeful way. However, Adams also reminds us that although the model may point the way to what must be learned about the dyslexic reader, and where we can begin to look for "dysfunctions, and weak, missing or misconstrued links", there is still much to be discovered.

Chapter 2:
The Dyslexic Learner

The dyslexic learner's most apparent difficulty is in learning to read. We expose young children to a variety of experiences, and somehow the ability to read becomes automatic, as automatic as speaking. When a child is offered the usual educational experiences, and fails to learn to read, we try to find explanations. We can observe that bright, curious, alert children with good language backgrounds learn to read more quickly and more efficiently than slow learners with limited language experience. Thus it is easy to assume that reading failure might be caused by inadequate parents, who have given poor language experience. Another common assumption is that the poor readers must be slow learners. In fact, it could be true that it is possible to be dyslexic, to have a poor language background, and to be a slow learner. If such a cluster of problems exists, diagnosis becomes a tricky business. The pattern of dyslexic difficulties is much easier to spot when the young learner is bright and knowledgeable, well motivated, and reared with its quota of nursery rhymes, story books and adult attention. The child who has difficulties in learning to read has become an urgent focus of attention, and we need to explore the reasons for an individual's failure, and to find ways of teaching to overcome the problem.

For the teacher interested in the changing views of the general nature of the problem, useful reviews abound (see Hulme and Snowling, 1994; Miles and Miles, 1990; Snowling and Thomson, 1991; the Introduction in Thomson and Watkins, 1990). Dyslexia has been seen as a neurological problem (Hinshelwood, 1917, Orton, 1925, 1937), or as a visual deficit (Rayner and Pollatsek, 1987). It has been seen as an educational or sociological problem (Burt, 1937). Its genetic and neuro-biological link is currently being examined (DeFries, 1991; Duane, 1991). Psychologists and linguists have been examining evidence that describes dyslexia as a linguistic coding defect and consensus is developing on a view of dyslexia as a phonological deficit, developmental in nature (see Hulme and Snowling, 1994; also Miles and Miles, 1990, chapter 9 for a simple review). The various inquiries have made contributions, both large and small, to an understanding of dyslexia.

Teachers are becoming increasingly aware that the dyslexic difficulty is more than a problem in learning to read. For some older learners, spelling, handwriting or fluent written self-expression can be seen as the major problem. Difficulties with spoken language are often less obvious, but as we look at literacy as a language process, we begin to bring them into focus. Most dyslexic learners have a history of unusual language development, many have had speech therapy as infants, and many continue to show signs of unusual ways of processing language. An individual may have a lively mind and good problem-solving abilities; but these are not much help in building in the neurological responses necessary for swift, fluent reading and writing. For this, you need good phonological awareness, an ability to quickly process speech, and an awareness of the minute differences in sounds.

At this point it might be helpful to examine a real child, who presents many (though not all) of the features found in dyslexic learners.

Language Difficulties of the Dyslexic Learner: Hugh's Story

Hugh was born after a problem-free pregnancy and delivery. He was a healthy child. He never crawled, but pulled himself upright on the furniture, walking confidently by the time he was 1 year old. He was late in beginning to talk, and had an unusual pattern of language development. He was a quiet baby. He laughed and cried, and shouted for attention, but made very few of the experimental babbling sounds that come from many infants. At the age of 15 months, he began to use cryptic one word utterances, usually nouns, leaving those around him to interpret the meaning. He gradually increased the length of his utterances, but spoke slowly and deliberately, and often had to grope for words. His receptive language seemed normal, and he enjoyed listening to stories and rhymes appropriate to his age. He could not pronounce initial 'r' until he began school, and substituted 'w'; otherwise, his articulation was clear.

On starting school, it was obvious that there were areas of difficulty that would make it hard for him to satisfy expectations. His clothes had to be chosen carefully, he could not tie bows in his shoe laces, and would sometimes forget halfway through whether or not he was dressing or undressing, and would begin to reverse the process. The days seemed endless to him, because he could neither tell the time (analogue or digital) nor sense where he was in the day. He could not learn the order of the days of the week, or associate each day with its appropriate activities.

Intellectually, he was making excellent progress, and asked searching questions about the world around him. He was a logical thinker, and enjoyed Maths, although he found it very difficult to remember number bonds. He could 'read' the flash cards when they had words and pictures, but wondered how the other children could still say the words when the teacher took the pictures away. By the time he was aged 7, he was aware of the growing gap between his achievement and that of his classmates, and was very unhappy at school. His self-esteem was further damaged by his younger sister's evident reading ability.

Despite considerable individual help, he failed to make progress in reading and writing, and was assessed by an educational psychologist at the age of 9. His reading level was two years behind his chronological age, and his spelling level, three years behind. His scores on the tests of the Weschler Intelligence Scales for Children (Revised) (WISC-R) placed him on the high average scales for IQ (Full Scale Score 118). His score on the WISC-R sub-tests showed a typically dyslexic profile (Thomson, 1984). He was very successful on tests that required good visual perception, spatial and constructional abilities, and scored at the superior level; however, his poor scores were on the subtests Arithmetic, Coding, Information and Digit span (the 'ACID' profile), all tests that tap verbal sequential memory.

On the advice of the psychologist, Hugh was referred to a communication therapist. She found that he had a word-finding difficulty: although he had a good receptive vocabulary, he could not easily retrieve the word he wanted. This difficulty spilled over into reading: although he could identify a hare from a group of pictures that included a rabbit, he could not retrieve the name in an illustrated text. He read "The hare ran across the field" as "The...., no, not a rabbit... the.... I can't remember what you call it... ran across the field". Each time, he was given the word, he repeated it, but had forgotten it on the next page. It is not surprising that 'association units', linking the letters on the page with appropriate sounds, were not being stored in his memory in a way that would enable quick recognition or recall.

Word-Finding Difficulties

'Children pick up words like a magnet picks up pins—possibly over ten a day' (Aitchison, 1987). By the time a child is 6 years old, its passive vocabulary could be 14 000 words (Carey, 1978). These words need to be accessed both for recognition and understanding, and for recall and use. To understand why the dyslexic child so often can be strong in recognition and yet so weak in recall, we need to look at the different aspects of word storage.

Hugh's most obvious problem was in the establishment of accurate phonological representation of words. *Content* and *use* of language (see Lahey's model p. 5) were relatively problem free, so that he could respond well to language that he heard, absorbing ideas and meanings. As he grew older, he found ways of disguising his poor word-finding ability. He made liberal use of words like 'thingy' and 'whatcher call it', and learned to encourage his conversational partner to supply the missing words. He was also a good social communicator, getting on well with other children and enjoying good relationships with adults. However, the sounds he stored were often 'fuzzy', and it was as if a new word had to carve out its own niche in the memory—there were no clearly marked, distinctive sound slots into which they could be quickly fitted. An anecdote from Hugh's infancy (he was aged 3) illustrates the problem.

Hugh's mother reported that Hugh had been taken to see a neighbour who kept hens, and was very interested in the whole experience. He fed them corn, and asked what else they could eat. He was fascinated to know that they produced eggs—one of his favourite foods—and he asked questions for weeks after about the genesis of the food on his plate. He noticed their likeness to other birds, and wanted to know if they could fly like the garden birds, or swim like the ducks in the park, or talk like his Aunt's budgie.

Although he could not recall the word 'duck' he knew how the word could be used correctly in speech. His substitutions were always nouns, and fitted correctly into his brief sentences.

The hen was fitted into an elaborate meaning web. Hugh had a lively interest in natural history, and understood the function of the hen, and its connection with the rest of his world. He knew it was a bird, neither wild nor a pet. But he could not remember the word 'hen', and called them "them birds in her garden", or "duts" (ducks), or "budgie". He had immediate recognition of the word, so some aspects of his phonological storage were effective. His problems manifested themselves when he was required to recall the word, and to match it quickly with the movements of mouth, tongue and breath so that he could say it.

In the Classroom

Teachers working with children like Hugh often find it difficult to justify their feeling that such pupils have a specific problem, and are not simply slow learners—they can't read, can't write, and may give garbled accounts of experiences. Evidence can be scanty, they just have a feeling that such pupils have wide interests and general knowledge, but that these are not reflected in their everyday class work. It is obvious that they understand more than they can record, and the poor written work is often cited as a reason for anxiety in the dyslexic child who has managed to develop enough reading ability to get by in the classroom. Poor handwriting and spelling skills are usually seen as the cause of the problem. But if you listen to what these children actually say, you may find that their spoken accounts are garbled and confused. They have the knowledge and understanding to build a picture for their listener, but when note is made of what they actually say, it can be surprising how much they manage to force their conversational partner to contribute to the conversation. Specific expressive weaknesses are often found in children's spoken language, although their wide general knowledge and good understanding allows them to mask these problems: they can give the impression that their problems are limited to written language. An approach that concentrates too narrowly on literacy skills will not be enough—the language problems have also to be addressed.

Sam, a boy aged 11, had such problems. He had never been thought of as a boy with language difficulties. His manners were formal and polite, and his speech was clear. His class teachers commented that he talked too much, and demanded more than his share of attention. Sam did not feel that his reading was a major problem, and his comprehension level was at about the 9;6 year level, enough for functional literacy. Writing was his major problem—he never wrote enough, and as soon as he concentrated on expression, his spelling and writing deteriorated. The sample below (figure 2.1) indicates the struggle: Sam was asked to write something about himself and his family for a new teacher. It took him 35 minutes, and he needed constant encouragement.

My farit 'hobey is Rgb and i like wood wurk my dad was a carf printer and an army man and hey was a ship yard man hes chus bedrngs now he yoss to wurkal at sligl sily

'My favourite hobby is rugby and I like woodwork my dad was a carpenter and an army man and he was a shipyard man he checks buildings now he goes to work at Steel City.'
Figure 2.1 Sam's free writing

Although Sam spoke quickly and apparently fluently, there were frequent little pauses, filled by facial tics accompanied by little audible squeaks. Unless his listeners were familiar with the background of his conversation, it was hard to disentangle the meaning, and it often took two or three questions to establish a joint context. A conversation with Sam was recorded and transcribed. Sam knew that the talk was being recorded, and he chose the topic: he wanted to talk about a coming performance of a school play.

S. (Sam): Well, Mrs X and Mrs Y are doing this play, and she asked us to put our hands up who wants to read a part, I put my hand up for one of, for Joseph, and I put it down without Miss seeing it, because I didn't really want to do Joseph, because I knew I wouldn't get it, and remember the seven sons, you had Benjamin in it.

T: (Teacher): Oh yes?

S: So I wanted to go to Benjamin.

T: Yes?

S: So I thought, said to Matt, You'll probably get Joseph and I'll probably get Benjamin, and Mum... When I told Mum and I said Benjamin went to the second sack out for the feast in the Bible, and Benjamin they would recognize him and its a bit upsetting when they paid money for him to get, to get lost and they got the coat.

T: The coat?

S: The coat of, the coat of many colours. They gave it back to Dad with some blood, some sheep blood on, no some goat blood on it.

T: Why did they do that?

S: Because they didn't 'cos they settled for second best 'cos they felt really jealous that he was getting all the praise.

Imagine trying to sort that out without previous knowledge of the story of Joseph. Is it surprising that Sam finds it difficult to focus on salient details in writing? Such children will find it helpful to have an assessment from a communication therapist, who will be able to identify specific problems and give useful advice to teachers responsible for constructing an Individual Educational Programme.

The chapter on assessment (p45) will help teachers decide on such a referral.

It is not uncommon for a beginner reader to substitute a familiar word for an unknown one, even if the letters are quite different. The child who read "What a horrible child you are!" when the text said "What a disgusting child you are!" was using good language skills, and a good knowledge of high-frequency words, to access meaning. Gradually, as phonic links develop, the good reader reacts accurately to the letters and letter clusters, thus increasing their knowledge of phonic links. But consider the child who looked at a box with the name 'Fox' on it, and said "That boy's called Wolf". Consider the adult who looked at the word 'burial' printed in a context-free word list, and said, "That's ..er...to do with Vernon's Undertakers". It is as if they are dipping into a different area of word storage, going straight into meaning, and missing out sound associations completely. It is easy to see the likely effects of inefficient phonological recall on the acquisition of literacy skills. Approaches to teaching reading and writing must take such weaknesses into account.

Chapter 3:
The Development of
Literacy Skills

How do children learn to read and write? Our own experiences influence our understanding. Some of us cannot remember how we learned. Reading came so easily to us that it seemed as natural a process as growing. Those of us who experienced early difficulties will remember vividly the hurt and anxiety resulting from failure, and perhaps the gratitude when a teacher found a key that helped to make things plain.

How we approach the teaching of reading and writing depends on what we see as natural development. Much of the recent research is practical, positive and helpful, and is giving us valuable clues in trying to find ways of helping children with reading and writing problems. Some of it concentrates on looking at successful readers, and asks how do they succeed?

A Staged Model

A helpful model was constructed by a psychologist, Uta Frith (1985). Looking carefully at the way children read and write, she describes three stages of literacy development.

Stage 1: Logographic

At this stage, children recognize a small but growing vocabulary of whole words. They look at a word as if it were a logo, or a picture. They respond to written language as though it were Chinese—that is, one word, one picture (Ellis, 1984). They can only read familiar words, in familiar contexts, in a familiar script. In writing, they might introduce a whole word, like their name, or a shop sign.

Some learners can give the impression that their writing is at the logographic stage when in fact they are making quite a lot of phonic attempts. At first sight, the sample below looks bizarre, but when you read the 'translation' you can see that Emma is moving towards the alphabetic stage: most of the words attempt sound symbol links. Once you eliminate b/d reversals, most of the boundary consonants are phonically represented, albeit inefficiently.

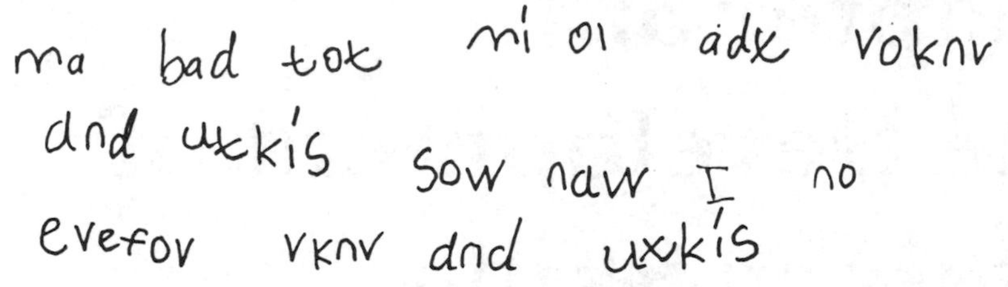

ma bad tok ni oi adx voknv
dnd uxki's sow naw I no
eveFov vknv dnd uxki's

'My Dad taught me all about volcanoes and earthquakes so now I know everything about volcanoes and earthquakes.

Figure 3.1 Emma's free writing

Stage 2: Alphabetic

Children seem to need to link sounds and letters together for spelling before they use the sound links for reading. They begin to 'invent' spellings; look at the example below (figure 3.2) typed onto the computer by a child aged 6. Nicholas's errors reflect his increasing sound awareness and letter knowledge. He is logically representing the consonant sounds (a biscuit: absct). His growing knowledge of letter names enables him to 'invent' a spelling for 'half' in which the name 'r' is used to represent the grapheme 'ar', and even for the whole word 'are'. Using this same technique, he can make a sensible attempt at 'Wendy'', using the letter name 'd' to represent the spoken syllable. He has learned a few whole words; for example, he can spell his own name. However, his ability to communicate is not held up while he finds the correct spelling for each word.

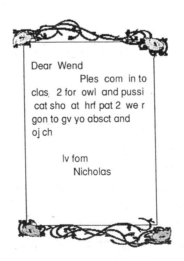

Dear Wend
            Ples com in to
clas 2 for owl and pussi
cat sho at hrf pat 2 we r
gon to gv yo absct and
oj ch

        lv fom
        Nicholas

'Dear Wendy
Please come into Class 2 for owl and pussy cat show at half past 2 we are going to give you a biscuit and orange juice.
love from Nicholas.'

Figure 3.2 Nicholas's letter

"The Flud" (figure 3.3) is an example from an older child. Rachel (aged 9) is able to use her mastery of basic sound–symbol links to communicate fluently. Indeed, her use of language is consciously literary, and she demonstrates use of deliberate graphic conventions in her use of capitals and punctuation. She can certainly read the word "flood", but the visual image of the word does not come back to her when she is writing. She has made a start in remembering whole words, but even a very commonly encountered phrase, 'Once upon a time', is only partially mastered. The only 'bizarre' spellings are the result of reversed letters (e.g. 'dey' for 'be').

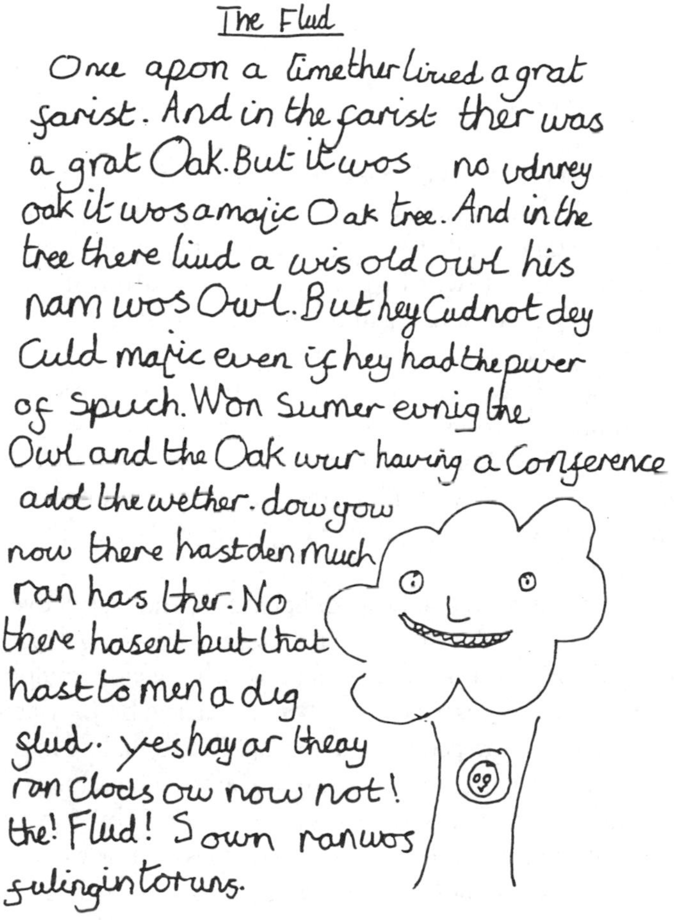

The Flud

Once apon a timether lived a grat
farist. And in the farist ther was
a grat Oak. But it wos no vdnrey
oak it wos a majic Oak tree. And in the
tree there liud a wis old owl his
nam wos Owl. But hey cudnot dey
Culd majic even if hey had the puver
of Speuch. Won Sumer evnig the
Owl and the Oak wur having a Conference
add the wether. dow you
now there hast den much
ran has ther. No
there hasent but that
hast to men a dig
slud. yes hay ar theay
ran Clods ow now not!
the! Flud! Sown ranwos
fulingintoruns.

'Once upon a time there lived a great forest. And in the forest there was a great Oak. But is was no ordinary oak, it was a magic Oak tree. And in the tree there lived a wise old owl his name was Owl. But he could not be called magic even if he had the power of speech. One summer evening the Owl and the Oak were having a conference about the weather. Do you know there hasn't been much rain has there. No there hasn't but that has to mean a big flood. Yes here are the rain clouds Oh no not! the! Flood! Soon rain was falling in torrents.'

Figure 3.3 Rachel's 'The Flud'

As the knowledge of letter–sound links grows, the skills begin to be transferred to reading. The child begins to respond first to initial sounds, and may then begin to 'sound out' unfamiliar words.

Stage 3: Orthographic

At this stage the child has internalized the traditional spelling patterns, and can recognize the elements that make up the words of the English language. They begin to recognize familiar suffixes and prefixes, and can break up a long word like 'unhopefully' by seeing the separate pieces (un-hope-ful-ly) rather than trying to tackle it letter by letter. Words begin to be read by analogy; when the word 'bread' is familiar, they can read the word 'spread'. At this stage, fluent reading does not inevitably ensure spelling proficiency (Fischer, 1985); abstraction of the rules, at a conscious or unconscious level, is also required in order to spell words like hoping/hopping.

Uta Frith suggests that dyslexic learners do not develop the ability to make quick and automatic links between letters and their sounds; they become arrested at the logographic stage. They have particular difficulty in acquiring alphabetic strategies—'sounding out' words does not come naturally. For reading, they depend on a small sight vocabulary, and use their knowledge of language to guess the rest. For writing, they often limit their output to the words they can spell, and use various strategies to accumulate the words they don't know, asking someone, finding words round the room, producing an artistic impression of the word, or not writing at all. With skilful teaching and hard work the well-motivated student can compensate for cognitive difficulties. But the development is not easy or natural. Frith, Shankweiler and Liberman (1992) recognise the "near superhuman effort" required.

The Frith model has proved to be an enlightening and instructive way of looking at the difficulties of such children, and of formulating teaching programmes to help them. Their need to focus on skills, perhaps at a very simple alphabetic level, is recognized. This model is described clearly in an article by Joy Stackhouse (1990). She describes a stage that precedes the logographic one, calling it 'pre-literate', and recognizing early writing attempts as communicative. The authors prefer the term 'emergent writing'; this term responds to the intention behind the attempts rather than judging the end product in terms of correctness. Thus we are reacting as we would to the early spoken language of the young infant, regarding it as an immature form of the more mature language that will develop later. We use also the positive term 'emergent reading' to describe the early stages of learning to read.

Emergent Literacy

Emergent reading

As well as interpreting the alphabetic code, the young reader and writer needs to develop a more general understanding of how written language, books and stories work. Marie Clay (1972, 1979) uses the phrase "concepts about print" to describe this. Emergent readers and writers develop this understanding through watching and listening to the adults around them and then imitating what they see and hear. Through their early experiences of print in the environment, such as labels on groceries, road signs, mummy's shopping list and birthday cards, and through sharing picture story books, the young child begins to learn that print carries a message.

Being read to is an important part of literacy development. It widens the child's experience of how books and stories work and brings the author's voice and language alive. The emergent reader learns that there is a correct way to hold a book, and that print has directional movement across a page. Books that have been shared with an adult will be returned to and 'read' again when the child is alone. The child retells the story through the pictures and the memory of the adult reading. The child's own ability to construct and understand a narrative through play and through talk is an essential part of this process. At this stage there is no exact match between the child's words and the words on the page. The results can be most entertaining, especially if the adult voice and actions are imitated too!

Gradually the aspects of the code become more familiar and the child's understanding becomes more sophisticated as the differences between words, letters, numbers, punctuation and sentences become clearer. Learning that written language can be used in this way to transmit messages, news, stories or rhymes is an important discovery, and we should not assume that the child entering school has understood this fully. Many children have had a limited experience in this area, or have been unable to make sense of their experiences.

As understanding of written language grows, the child begins to interpret aspects of print more consistently and moves into the logographic stage of reading.

Emergent writing

Emergent writing develops in a similar way to reading. The child observes adults writing and then imitates them. Early writing attempts where the young child explores the conventions of letter shapes and of writing have been likened to the babble and articulatory practice of a young child exploring speech sounds. During this early stage, however, there are no direct links between the letter shapes and the speech they represent. Early explorations may involve imitation of the different aspects of writing that children notice, from the writing of specific letter-like shapes to the reams of linear marks that some children produce in imitation of the speed, direction and flow that they see when adults write.

In early childhood, drawings and writing are produced together. The drawings are as much a part of the total message or idea as that which may be distinguished separately as writing. Drawing conventions or signs are established that represent, for example, houses or faces. As more forms that are distinguishable as writing begin to emerge, there is further tangible evidence of the growing ability to represent thought symbolically.

Very young children's writing may consist of marks that do not seem to look like letters or pictures but are representational in some other way. Whitehead (1990) refers to a young child's marks that attempt to imitate the movement and personal feelings held towards a family pet rather than a graphic image of the cat itself. Such representations have to be experienced along with the child for them to be correctly interpreted!

Gradually the young writer moves towards more letter-like shapes and conventions and towards the logographic stage.

Claire's writing of her own name and of Mummy (figure 3.4) includes a combination of pictures, linear marks and some letter-like shapes. All are written from left to right following the conventions of print that Claire has observed.

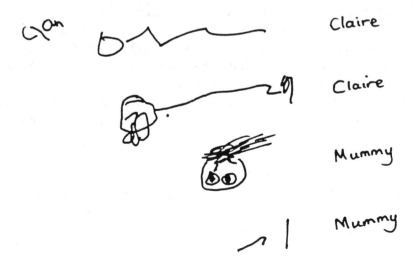

Figure 3.4 Claire's writing

Martyn's first piece of writing (figure 3.5) was made in response to his observations of another child writing lists of the names of children in his class. There is a definite M for Martyn in the bottom left hand corner along with other marks, stabs and lines.

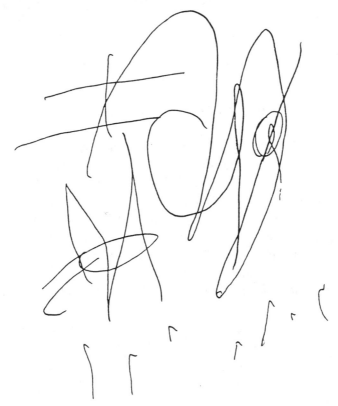

Figure 3.5 Martyn's writing

The second piece (figure 3.6) was made several months later in response to a request to write a story. The format of the four picture sequence was suggested by the teacher.

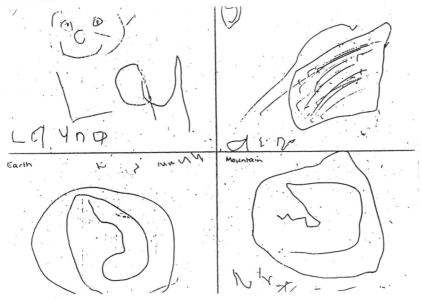

Figure 3.5 Martyn's picture-story

The story reads as follows:

picture 1: Laura
picture 2: went in a rocket
picture 3: to earth
picture 4: and climbed a mountain.

Martyn successfully uses pictures, letter shapes and representational marks to write his story. Notice the 'whoosh' of the rocket in picture 2 represented by dramatic strokes of the pencil (and sound effects!). His pictures of the earth as seen from space are effective and are accompanied by left to right text. Note also the mountains in the middle of the earth in picture 4.

Although at an early stage in their writing, both Martyn and Claire show that they have understood a great deal about the conventions of print and its representational nature. For a more detailed study of early writing development see Clay's (1975) *What Did I Write?*, which takes us through the different principles and stages that emerge.

Young children also notice the writing formats that adults use and may produce lists and letters to family members similar to those produced by the adults around them. Children in nursery and reception classes take great delight in writing such messages to their teachers, and open access to writing materials (see p.67) can facilitate this. David, a young dyspraxic child in a special school, would make diaries out of card and paper, and make his own entries as he had seen his teacher do. His diary, like hers, had an elastic band round the cover, with messages and reminder notes slipped inside. David's writing consisted of linear marks and some letter-like shapes, but he could tell the message behind them. He would also make registers in the same way.

At the emergent stage of writing the child discovers the first links between spoken and written language. It is recognized that print carries a message and the child explores this discovery. As teachers of learners at this stage of development we should be concerned with the process of writing rather than the correctness of the handwriting, spelling or grammar. It is where the foundations of later literacy are laid and is as important for the older learner with reading difficulties as for the younger child following the usual pattern of development. The older learner may be more inhibited and less productive, knowing, for example, that spellings can be 'wrong'. The younger child, less aware of such judgments, is more relaxed and adventurous.

Chapter 4:
Phonological Awareness

The English language, like most modern writing systems, has an alphabetic code. Letters represent sounds. The match between letter and sound, though to some extent inconsistent, is generally reliable. On meeting print, the child is able to map letters onto sounds already stored for spoken language. The child who has stored good, clear, explicit phonological representations is going find it much easier to make the links necessary for fluent reading and writing. Development of sound awareness affects reading and writing skills; in turn, sound awareness is affected by increasing reading ability. Success in this process depends heavily on the integrity of the sounds stored for spoken language. Fuzzy representations of sounds can lead to strange mistakes in spoken language. John (aged 9) was half listening to a conversation about his teacher's 'peripatetic' role; he wondered if she was called a 'very pathetic' teacher because she had to be so kind to her pupils. He drew attention to a 'jack hammer', and told his teacher that its real name was a 'dramatic' (pneumatic) drill. At this stage John had no obvious communication difficulties, his speech appeared fluent and clear, though he had problems in acquiring clear articulation of new vocabulary. He wanted a 'mocatrow' car for Christmas, and was enchanted to see the strange playground words written down as 'remote control'. As soon as he was shown the written syllables, he could map onto them the string of sounds and gain insight into the meaning. Such children, often with a history of speech and language difficulties, find it hard to move smoothly into being fluent readers and writers.

When we are speaking or listening, attention is focused on meaning. We do not need conscious awareness of words, syllables and sounds for talking and listening. For reading and writing, the learner has to become aware of these sub-units. Moreover, explicit awareness of sounds is predictive of future reading ability. We will examine the normal development of sound awareness, and think about its links with reading and writing.

Pattern of Development

Awareness of Words and Syntax

In connected speech we do not necessarily make clearly identified breaks between what we as adults understand to be words. Our words often run into each other in a continuous stream of sound patterns and yet we still know the individual words are there.

Research into children's concept of 'words' as linguistic entities has shown that although there may be some awareness of content words (nouns, adjectives, and verbs) before formal schooling, this develops further once reading begins (see Ehri, 1979).

Initially in word learning there is a focus of attention on meaning. This may cause difficulty in separating words from phrases; for example, 'big dog' may be understood as one word. The word 'train' may be understood to be a long word because trains are long, or the word 'ladybird' may be thought to be a little word because ladybirds are little. Function words, such as 'is' and 'the', which bind the meaning in our sentences together, may not be recognized as words as they do not have easily identified meanings. Poor reading ability can mean that dyslexic learners stay confused for years, leading to errors such as 'Sheffeel Junited', 'an ife' (a knife). Once literacy begins, children attend to individual words more easily and begin to move closer to the adult's concept of 'word'.

In the same way that meaning affects the concept of 'word', the acceptability of the meaning of a sentence may affect a child's view of its grammatical correctness (Tunmer and Bower, 1984). This acceptability may depend on personal experience. For example, "Daddy cooked the dinner" may not be considered correct if mummy always cooks. Conversely, a grammatically incorrect sentence may not be noticed if there is meaning for the child, for example, "the dog runned away".

Both the development of word and syntactical awareness have great significance for reading and writing. Children can use this developing knowledge to help with the decoding of unfamiliar words and in self-correction of errors. However, until a more mature awareness of words and syntax develops we will still encounter the child who reads 'big dog' for 'dog'. For this child, the understanding of the concept overrides other information that they might be receiving from the print on the page.

Awareness of Syllables

Words are spoken in syllables, each syllable being formed by a push of air from the lungs. This strong physical basis for syllable formation in speech production makes it easy to alert pre-school children to syllables in speech (Liberman *et al.*, 1974; Treiman and Baron, 1981). But syllables are even further removed from meaning than words, so conscious awareness of them is harder to acquire. Some of the most bizarre spellings we come across are attempts at multisyllabic words, where some of the consonant sounds are desperately scattered onto the page. Coming across a long word in print can be too daunting to attempt.

Awareness of Phonemes (Speech Sounds)

A phoneme is the smallest unit of sound that changes a spoken word. Normal development results in an acute sensitivity to minute differences in words, so that 'but' is not pronounced in the same way as 'put', and 'bag' does not sound exactly the same as 'back'. Young children are not consciously aware of making these fine discriminations, just as they are not aware of the sophisticated and elaborate movements required for them to be able to neatly spoon yogurt into their mouths. They have a working knowledge of phonemes, not a conscious one. Young children, though expert at using fine differences to interpret and express meaning in talk, cannot use this skill in conscious analysis, and they perform poorly on tasks that require them to identify the single phonemes of a word or syllable (Bruce, 1964; Liberman et al., 1974).

Frith (1985) asserts that children first move from logographic stage to alphabetic for spelling rather than reading, and teachers find that young children first become interested in phonemes when they want to express themselves in writing. Finding that you can 'invent' your own spellings facilitates free communication, and Charles Read (1986) lists some fascinating examples—try reading these aloud if you are not quite sure what they mean:

Tom nicta cr
My Dadaay wrx hir
B cwiyit.

Awareness of Onset and Rime: an Intermediate Stage

Some tasks that require awareness of phonemes are easier than others. Babies and toddlers demonstrate a working knowledge of rhyme and alliteration. They delight in experimental sound play, including the repetition of syllables that have the same beginning (alliteration) or the same ending (rhyme). Chukovsky (1963) asserts that the making of rhymes is an essential part of normal development in the second year of life. Such spontaneous word games are 'linguistic exercises'. Before children go to school, their knowledge of rhyme can be explicit— many of them can make judgments about which words rhyme (Dowker, 1989; Read, 1971). They can also detect the 'odd one out' in a list like 'ham, had, tap, hat' (Bradley and Bryant, 1983), a task requiring awareness of alliteration. Linguists have developed their view of phonemic development, and are interested in the natural tendency in all languages for speakers to be sensitive to divisions they describe as onset and rime. Goswami and Bryant (1990) describe this as an 'intermediate kind of phonological awareness', falling between sensitivity to syllables and sensitivity to individual sounds. Until recently, the syllable was regarded within the field of linguistics as a linear string of phonemes (e.g. Hooper, 1972):

frog: /f/ /r/ /o/ /g/   pen: /p/ /e/ /n/

A two syllable word first divides into syllables, then each syllable into phonemes:

magnet mag: /m/ /a/ /g/   net: /n/ /e/ /t/

The view most widely accepted by current linguistic theory is that the syllable has a natural division into two major sub-units, onset and rime. The onset is the initial consonant or consonant cluster. The rime is the vowel, and anything that comes after.

Table 4.1 Intrasyllabic Units

Word	Syllable	Onset and rime	Phoneme
dot	dot	d - ot	d -o -t
swing	swing	sw - ing	s - w - i - ng
cobweb	cob - web	c - ob w - eb	c- o - b - w - e -b

Onset and rime are the most salient units within a language, the bits that are manipulated in 'secret' languages and word games. Pinker (1994) reminds us of 'pig Latin', and 'Yinglish' constructions such as 'fancy-shmancy', 'Oedipus-shmoedipus' where words are spliced at the onset–rime boundary. Natural mistakes such as 'spoonerisms' ('par cark' for 'car park', 'the queer old dean' for 'the dear old queen') use the onset and rime division. Many children can perform onset and rime tasks before they start to read (Maclean, Bryant and Bradley, 1987; Treiman and Zukowski, 1991), and Goswami (1986) found that children were consistently more successful in using analogies that divided words at the onset–rime division. (i.e. 'eak' in beak, peak, weak, rather than 'bea' in bean, bead, beat). They certainly find these tasks easier than those that require appreciation of single phonemes, especially if they are required to recognize the first sound of a consonant cluster. Research into the phonemic awareness of illiterate adults supports these findings. In Britain, which has a long history of universal education, most adults have had reading experience, but in some countries it has been possible to compare the phonemic awareness of groups who have been introduced to reading and those who have not. Goswami and Bryant (1990) review the research on phonological processing and reading ability, and put forward a convincing account of the theory that rhyme and alliteration are skills that learners bring to the task of reading; phoneme detection is a skill that develops as written language is introduced, and develops along with literacy skills. (Treiman, 1992; see Bertelson and de Gelder, 1989 for a review).

Implications for Reading

For younger readers, sensitivity to sound and phonic knowledge are good predictors of future reading ability, and are more important than cognitive functioning (see Adams, 1990). She reviews the weighty body of evidence suggesting that awareness of the speech sounds within words and knowledge of letter names are the two strong predictors of early reading progress. More recently, a study carried out by McDougall and Hulme (1994) confirmed these theories. They add the intriguing finding that speed at which familiar words can be articulated is also a factor in the development of reading. This further emphasizes the importance of the processing of spoken language in learning to read. When starting formal reading instruction, we must take into account the learner's stage of sound processing. Infants gradually acquire and refine their use of sound patterns in speech. As they babble, they map the speech they hear onto the sounds they make. Most children have a well formed sound system by the time they are expected to learn to read.

Skilled reading is an interactive process, depending on the spelling pattern of a word, its meaning, and its pronunciation. Adams (1990) describes how a skilled reader processes the individual letters of a text with impressive ease and speed, building up expectations about relationship between letters and sounds, which she calls 'association units'. Adult readers who have built these association units will find it hard to imagine what a page of print can look like to a learner who sees only lines of letters. We gain occasional insight from mistakes—like Owen, who asked if he could see any little words in the big one ('someone'), triumphantly produced 'so', 'me', and 'on', with a spare 'e'. The association units are beginning to be assembled, but there is still some way to travel.

The evidence linking progress in reading to underlying sound processing skills is impressive. There is some debate about the effects of different phonological abilities on literacy development: Goswami and Bryant (1990) feel that rhyming ability is the most important predictor, and Muter (1994) found that ability in phoneme segmentation is a better predictor of use of analogies at the ages of 5 and 6. A number of studies, plus a mass of evidence from the observations of the Reading Recovery teams of Marie Clay (1993a and b), suggest that phonological training should be combined with explicit instruction about letters and spelling patterns, and be rooted in the reading of real texts (see Hatcher, 1994).

Multisensory Teaching and Phonological Awareness

Traditional multisensory structured approaches (see p.36) that have been used for teaching dyslexic children require modification, and must take into account phonological awareness. With Frith's stages in front of us, we can endeavour to move the child from logographic techniques to alphabetic ones. Multisensory structured methods are an excellent tool for enabling the child to make this step. Dyslexic children can usually be taught to communicate by writing, using alphabetic techniques, and employing the most likely letter for each sound. (See 'The Flud', p.20—*grat / great; nam / name; cudnot / could not*).

However, although the ability to 'invent' spellings can enable the writer to communicate, reliance on logical letter sound matching will not lead to fluent reading. Until the reader has begun to make 'association units' that can coincide with traditional spelling patterns, efficient reading of normal, simple texts is not possible. In order to become fluent, the reader needs to recognize the *at* in cat, or the *ight* in night as whole units. Unless the child is going to be taught English as if it were a logographic language like Chinese, use of analogy must be encouraged as a futher step in decoding. Thus knowledge of *ight* can become a key to *flight*, *bright*, etc.

Training studies (Bruck and Treiman, 1992; Goswami, 1994) suggest that programmes of instruction should not focus only on individual phonemes, as traditional phonic programmes did. They should instead take note of the level of phonological skills available to the child on entry to school. In England, where children start formal education at the age of 5, they usually have onset and rime skills. Whilst working on the acquisition of a sound knowledge of name, sound, appearance and formation of each of the 26 letters of the alphabet, it is a good idea to encourage use of analogy, building on the natural verbal ability to divide syllables at the onset-and-rime boundary, and the ability to categorize words by sound.

The average child of 6 or 7 would find it difficult to handle the concepts that would enable it to read the word 'ice'. That simple word combines two common spelling rules—'magic e' and 'soft c', defying the rule that print is deciphered from left to right. But 'ice' is a word commonly found in print, usually along with 'cream'. Children with good ability to perceive rhyme may notice that 'nice price' have letters in common, and may also have sound in common. Knowledge of sounds and knowledge of spelling patterns influence each other as children focus on spelling sequences that correspond to rhymes. Increased familiarity with spelling patterns comes with increased reading experience and refined phonemic knowledge, which leads to awareness of letter–sound links.

Dyslexic learners, even those with excellent cognitive skills, can take years to realise that the English language is not a logographic one, and that generalities can be made. They are not going to use analogies spontaneously and easily, and often have surprising gaps at an alphabet level. Teaching methods must include phonemic training (Bruck and Treiman, 1992; Ehri and Robbins, 1992). The focus on phonemes is necessary for use of initial sound cues, and for invented spellings. The dyslexic learner will not readily absorb these links, and overlearning will be necessary before they become automatic, but the programme must also include specific training on observation of rime units. The learner needs to develop knowledge of rimes that provide important keys, and strategies in using them. The programme developed and described here closely integrates these elements, and takes into account the special characteristics and special needs of the dyslexic learner.

Chapter 5:
Teaching Reading

The approach to the teaching of reading used in this book is based on the view of dyslexia as a language disorder, on recent research into reading difficulties, and on a strong belief in an integrated approach to written language. To put our approach into context, it is first useful to look at more traditional approaches to the teaching of reading.

Some Common Approaches

The terms 'top down' and 'bottom up' are often used to try and explain the difference between reading approaches. 'Bottom up' refers to a process that starts at the level of the print on the page and moves upwards. The reader moves from decoding letters and words and works upwards to the meaning of the whole text. 'Top down' refers to the reader starting with the whole text, looking for meaning based on contextual clues and then using these to work down to the level of the print on the page. Such descriptions give a guide to the essential differences between traditional reading approaches. However, if we bear in mind the model put forward by Adams (1994) they are very simplistic views of the reading process. The main approaches used in schools that could be described as 'bottom up' are 'phonics' and 'look and say'. The 'top down' approaches are 'real books' and 'language experience'.

'Bottom Up' Approaches

'*Look and say*' requires the ability to learn and recognize whole words by their visual appearance. This is usually achieved through the use of a graded series of reading scheme books with carefully controlled and gradually increased vocabulary. It may also involve the use of flash cards, reading games and activities aimed at increasing sight vocabulary. These activities may even precede the reading of the book, ensuring that the child will be able to read the words before encountering them in the text. This approach uses a core of words accepted as most frequently occurring in written texts and in children's own reading and writing. These are also referred to as keywords or high frequency words.

The old style of reading schemes has been heavily criticized for being unappealing and for failing to reflect the child's real experience of the world. More recently introduced schemes such as the *Oxford Reading Tree*, and *Sunshine* readers, have addressed some of these difficulties.

Phonic approaches to the teaching of reading are based on knowledge of letter sounds. A hierarchy of skills is learned, based on the letter sound correspondences that make up written language. Once individual letter sounds are learned the child is encouraged to blend sounds together and attack unfamiliar words independently. Phonically based reading schemes, backed up by games and activities, offer texts with controlled vocabularies, limiting them to words that are mainly made up of the sounds that have been learned. 'Difficult' sounds are avoided; for example, some of the less common double vowel combinations, and soft 'c' and 'g', are often introduced in later books. Such simple, early texts can give confidence and encourage the learner to feel confidence in developing independent reading skills. The *New Way* series is an example of simple, enjoyable stories, using lots of short vowel words that a learner can decipher using limited sound blending skills. The books they replace (the old *Gayway* series) are an example of what to avoid—in those, the structure is tighter, but the language is stilted and artificial, with limited vocabulary, contrived story lines and grammatical constructions.

Texts can be even more carefully structured, and attempts have been made to provide reading material that limits the number of letters. Augur and Briggs (1992) in their revision of Hickey's book (1977) add more 'Stories for fun' to the original work, specifying that some of them are for reading only. The example here (p. 229) uses only 15 letters:

> 'The happy man stands on top of the bin. He hops and the bin spins.He has a spiky hat on. He is off to Penny's picnic.'It is sad Penny is not at the picnic yet,' he said.The tiny cat comes and sits by the man. It is Penny's cat. He is happy to sit with the cat at the picnic as he has not met anyone. He assists with the sticky candy and the pop. Then he sits with the cat as he has his snacks. In the end Penny comes and sits with the man. She pops his spiky hat on. He is Penny's Dad.'

Such contrived and restricted language hinders prediction, and encourages letter by letter decoding. Skilled reading demands flexibility and quick, automatic choice of a suitable strategy (see p.66). There are advantages to both phonic and look and say approaches. They have a clear structure to follow, and they usually have a wealth of back-up materials. Carefully graded texts may mean that the young reader is not exposed to books that are too difficult, but may result in the child, parent or teacher feeling that only reading scheme books should be read. Phonic approaches encourage decoding skills, and thus eventually independence. *Look and say* relies on learning and reading familiar words, and may not encourage independence. Through over-reliance on 'bottom up' approaches, there may be a tendency for children to develop mechanical reading skills without reading for meaning.

'Top Down' Approaches

Shared reading has also been called 'whole language', a 'story book' approach, 'apprenticeship' to reading, and 'real books'. It arose out of dissatisfaction with the mechanical emphasis of 'bottom up' approaches, and with the stilted language of reading schemes. The label 'real books' was coined to reflect the use of picture, story and information books rather than traditional reading schemes. The development of the theory behind shared reading sprang from research into how children acquired spoken language (see p.5) The importance of parents reading to their children and sharing books with them was recognized as having a positive effect on later reading development (Wells, 1986). Reading *with* someone rather than reading *to* them became an essential part of this approach, along with an emphasis on meaning and the use of contextual clues.

Don Holdaway (1979) is said to have introduced shared reading into our classrooms. He suggested that the books read to children and shared with them should become the texts used in their reading programmes. He suggested that children's familiarity with the texts might enable them to read them independently. The emphasis was on the active involvement of the child, and the adult as supportive guide. This approach is now an integral part of the Reading Recovery programme (Clay, 1993b).

Holdaway's approach describes different stages in the use of a story:

1.   Initial discovery—when the book is first introduced and read to the child. Depending on the confidence of the child and the accessibility of the text, this might also include some reading alongside the adult reader.
2.   Exploration of the text—through rereading, reading alongside the adult and through activities that relate to and arise out of the text. By rereading a known text a child is more able to predict the sense and the language.
3.   Independent experience and expression—where the text is reread independently or re-enacted. The level of teacher support obviously varies according to the familiarity of the book and the confidence and skill of the child. The learner is encouraged to take as active a role as possible and collaborate with the adult in reading the book. This might involve discussing the pictures, guessing what is going to happen next, reading alongside, filling in pauses and taking over when confident enough to do so. The adult is there to add further support and to take over the reading again if appropriate.

There is much to be gained from shared reading and the real books movement. However, the overzealousness of some of its advocates drew attention away from the teaching of phonic skills. Our studies of dyslexic readers point to the importance of phonological skills. We should therefore draw attention to the alphabetic code as we share books with our learners.

The '*language experience approach*' is frequently used with young children. It uses the child's own language as a starting point to dictate captions, stories and books, which are then read back. The adult acts as scribe and gradually helps the child to realise the requirements of a written text . The adult here works in a similar way to the adult scaffolder in shared reading. *Breakthrough to Literacy* (MacKay et al., 1978) extends the language experience approach, using word folders, stands for sentence making, and scheme books.

There are positive benefits to be gained from top down approaches as they help us focus on the purpose of reading—meaning. The language experience approach is child centred using the child's own language as a basis for further learning. The 'real books' used in shared reading can be highly motivating to the reader as they are less contrived than scheme books, have quality illustrations and their own literary style.

It is obvious that no one approach has all the answers. In reality, teachers frequently use a mix of methods but tend to rely more heavily on one particular approach according to their own or the school's philosophy. Many children learn to read easily no matter what type of approach is used. For others, the route to literacy is painful and slow. Work by Barr (1974) showed that the approaches adopted by teachers had a strong influence on the strategies used by the children. Despite this, the natural strengths of the learner were often ignored. Approaches used should take into account the individual profile of a learner's development. This becomes even more important for learners with special educational needs.

Traditional Reading Approaches and the Dyslexic Learner

We have referred to the link between literacy difficulties and speech and language problems (pp.7, 12). Case history notes of children referred with dyslexia often reveal previous speech and language difficulties. Sometimes the problems may have appeared slight—perhaps unclear speech that has not even warranted speech therapy. Children such as these may fail to learn from traditional phonic approaches because of their underlying phonological processing difficulties. They are unable to make the fine discriminations needed, and are slow to learn phoneme/grapheme correspondences. They find it difficult to segment words into syllables, and to blend sounds together. They may make some progress in reading through visual strategies, but continue to have difficulty with spelling.

Some struggling readers also seem to have vocabulary difficulties. It may be that they have a limited vocabulary, but there are also a significant number of learners like Hugh (p.13) who are unable to access or 'find' a word they want to use. The required word remains out of reach, despite its existence in the child's vocabulary, and one similar in meaning or sound is accessed instead. Alternatively, a descriptive phrase or generality such as 'thingy' may be used. In order to visually recognize or predict a word successfully, the word has to exist within the child's lexicon, and there has to be ready access to it. Reading approaches that emphasize instant word recognition, particularly out of context, are probably going to be unsuccessful. Even with appropriate contexts dyslexic learners are slow to acquire a sight vocabulary. Recent interest in the area of children with word finding difficulties suggests the roots of the problem may be complex. In order to be learned and retrieved, words have to be perceived, understood and stored correctly in the first place according to a combination of factors concerned with meaning, syntax and phonological information. Underlying phonological processing difficulties may mean that these connections are faulty. Such children may therefore also have difficulty using a phonic route to reading.

Most learners with special educational needs do not develop skills through discovery. They require a structured approach to facilitate their learning. Shared reading and language experience approaches do not always provide the degree of structure needed. Also, they may not provide the experiences needed to enable these struggling readers to break into the alphabetic code and become more independent.

There are aspects from both top down and bottom up approaches that are appropriate for the pupils we teach and these are included in our teaching programme. However, for those children that experience severe difficulty in learning to read, other approaches have been developed. They take into account the particular difficulties experienced by the dyslexic learner, and aim to compensate for specific weaknesses.

Special Approaches for the Dyslexic Learner

Multisensory Learning

Reading and writing are multisensory activities. The learner is required to look at print, and say (or subvocalize) sounds, then use language skills to access meaning. The child needs the ability to form automatic and permanent links between the print in front of the eyes, and the sounds that words make, and link these with the meaning. The reader is paying attention to messages received through the eyes and ears, and also through reinforcement from the bits of the body that say the words—the delicate distinctions between voiced and unvoiced sounds that are felt in the nerves and muscles of the lips, tongue, teeth and throat. Writing adds to the involvement of the arm and hand. To recognize, remember and write a single word involves the whole body; eyes, ears, touch and movement—neurons flash between the different parts of the brain that control these functions.

Most children learn written language in the same way as they learn spoken language; given normal exposure to printed material, in and out of the classroom, the brain can build into its networks the patterns that lead to relaxed, fluent reading and writing. Adams (1994) describes this process as 'automaticity'; the skilled reader recognizes words and phrases at an amazing speed, and with such ease that they can free their mind to attend to meaning, in the same way as a skilled typist can automatically strike the separate keys in the correct order, whilst concentrating on the formulation of the next bit of the sentence. Learning a physical activity such as dancing, driving or swimming gives insight into this process. At first, each small, precise action has to be learned, and we can verbalize and list the positioning and movements of bits of the body. As the actions become automatic, it can be difficult to explain to a new learner how these processes take place. Reading and writing are automatic, interactive processes; but they rest on the recognition of individual words and letters.

Multisensory structured teaching methods, which focus on the establishment of automatic links between sound and symbol have been developed, and can be a useful tool in establishing speedy and permanent mastery of some of the basic units of written language. We need to take on board the message that Thomson and Watkins (1990) spell out in capital letters: "THERE ARE MANY ROUTES TO THE SAME OBJECTIVE". The automatic, interactive process we are describing is essentially an individual one, and the adaptation of any teaching programme must take into account both the teacher and the learner. But that doesn't mean we all have to invent the wheel from scratch, and we can benefit from the experience of others. The important thing is to remember that the objective is not multisensory teaching from the teacher: the objective is multisensory learning within the learner.

Traditional Multisensory Structured Teaching Methods

Gillingham and Stillman pioneered these methods in the 1930s. They aimed to build into the learner 'linkages' between phonemes and graphemes (sounds and letter/s). Routines are established that take into account recognition and recall of phoneme/grapheme links. The routines allow the learner to accumulate the linkages gradually, and to exercise them daily, so that the memory of the links does not fade. The approach is basically phonetic—sound units taught are first phonemes represented by individual letters, moving onto sounds represented by two or more letters (e.g. th, ch, igh). Their *Red Book* (Gillingham and Stillman, 1969) is a detailed training manual, and their work has been a driving force behind most of the multisensory schemes adapted to the English educational scene. The most influential of these is Kathleen Hickey's *Dyslexia: A Language Training Course for Teachers and Learners* (1977), which has been comprehensively edited and updated by Jean Augur and Suzanne Briggs (1992). The letter order in this volume starts with the same letters as the *Red Book*, the Hickey Course, and the *Texas Scottish Rite Hospital Course for Language Therapists* (Cox, 1967).

The most distinctive feature of these programmes is their emphasis on the kinesthetic aspects of learning. Teachers habitually use audio-visual techniques to good effect; multisensory techniques also involve kinesthetic aspects of learning, integrating 'output' (say and write) with 'input' (hear and see). At each stage of the programme, careful attention is given to the sound made by the learner, and the links with the written form of the letter. The dyslexic learner is notoriously weaker at recall than recognition, but current research is beginning to focus specifically on weaknesses in expressive phonology rather than discrimination. (See Hulme and Snowling's (1992) account of the 'selective deficit of output phonology' suffered by JM, a developmental dyslexic. See also Hulme and Snowling (1994) for an account of the relationship between speech skills, verbal short-term memory, phonological awareness, and the acquisition of literacy).

Multisensory techniques have been used to enrich many thoughtful and eclectic programmes currently in use—*Alpha to Omega* (Hornsby and Shear, 1975), 'Beat Dyslexia' materials, The Bangor Programme (Cooke, 1993; Miles, 1992), and the excellent individualized programmes worked out for the pupils of East Court School (Thomson and Watkins, 1990). Some programmes based on spelling rules and Hickey's spelling choices are helpful for learners with mild spelling problems, but may start at a point well in advance of the dyslexic learner's phonological skill. Teaching a spelling choice is not a useful technique for a child still struggling with the sound values of initial letters.

Supportive Approaches for Children with Speech and Language Difficulties: Cued Articulation and Rebus Symbols

In addition to their literacy difficulties, some children have significant problems in articulation or in expressive or receptive language. It should be stressed that the help of a communication specialist must be sought in these cases. Two approaches that may give extra support are cued articulation and rebus symbols. Dyslexic learners can also benefit from these approaches. They find it helpful to use cued articulation to support them in building sound–letter links. Rebus symbols can help them in learning key vocabulary.

Cued Articulation (Passey, 1993) is a gestural system used by speech therapists to aid the perception, discrimination and production of speech sounds. One simple, logical gesture indicates how and where a sound is made. Movements and position of tongue and lips are indicated by the shape of the hand. For example, when we make the sound /p/ we close both lips, stopping the release of air; then we open our lips and the air is released with a slight push. The gesture that emulates this is made by holding the hand close to the mouth, pressing together the index finger and the thumb, and gently jerking them apart. The system helps the learner distinguish between subtle differences in sounds such as voicing and unvoicing. The gesture for /b/ has a second finger closed on the thumb with the index finger to indicate the strength of the voicing. Other voiced/voiceless pairs are distinguished in the same way with one finger for unvoiced sounds, two for voiced. The place where the sound is made in the mouth or throat is indicated by hand positions (e.g. the gestures for /k/ and/g/ are made in front of the throat; the gestures for /p/ and /b/ are made at the side of the mouth).

On first reading, the system may sound complicated, but it is very easy to master, both for teachers and learners. Buy Passey's (1993) little book. You will find it possible to follow without help, though five minutes with a speech therapist familiar with the system will save time. Passey also includes a system of underlining and colour coding for written symbols.

Cued articulation can be very helpful for learners who have no obvious problems in articulating sounds, but who get weak messages from the sounds they make. They tend to make spelling errors (e.g. 'cow' for 'go') that reflect confusion between pairs of voiced and unvoiced sounds. The gestures help illustrate the similarities and differences in these sounds. The transient nature of spoken language can cause problems for some learners attempting to improve their spelling. The addition of a visual sign can be extremely helpful. Cued articulation makes the learning truly multisensory as the learner focuses on the gesture, the feel of the sound in the voice and the throat, the letter they see and write, and the sound they hear.

Cued articulation can also be a short cut in teaching. It cuts out verbal explanations dealing with the difference between /f/, /v/ and /th/, or /p/ and /b/. The gestures themselves demonstrate the difference—a boon to learners with weak auditory sequential memory. A learner with poor sound awareness can find that the sign actually teaches them that certain difficult sounds exist. Until we used cued articulation, most learners could only cope with the phonemes such as /ks/ in six, /ng/ in sting and /ngk/ in tank if they were presented as part of a rime. With the use of cued articulation, we find that most learners can conceptualize those sounds, and say them quite easily.

Rebus symbols are pictorial representations of spoken or written words. Each symbol represents a whole word. Pictures representing nouns are generally understood without explanation. Other words are less easily represented; function words are, on the whole, logical, but need some explanation.

Have a look at some examples:

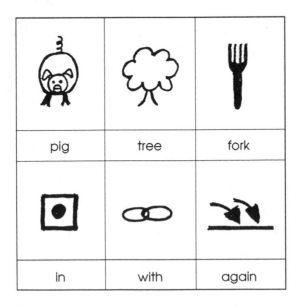

Figure 5.1 Rebus symbols

Additional symbols to indicate grammatical inflections such as tense markers or comparatives are also part of the system.

Rebus symbols have been traditionally used as an aid to spoken communication for those with communication disorders, or as an aid to concept development for individuals with more general or severe learning difficulties. However, they have also been used for some time to teach reading. It is thought that words that are associated with pictures might be more easily learned. For learners with communication problems rebuses are better than little drawings that the teacher might produce spontaneously. A child with word finding difficulties may be storing the words *dog, fox* and *wolf* under the same visual image and may have to grope for the correct label, and needs to be presented with a consistent image for each word. The symbols have been standardized and are constantly evolving. The LDA rebus glossary (Van Oosteroom and Devereux, 1992) contains an up-to-date list of about a thousand words. The teacher can use it for tracing and copying, and it can also serve as a picture dictionary for older learners who find that dictionaries with picture clues designed for younger learners are too immature for their liking. Makaton symbols have recently been extended to include words related to the National Curriculum Programme of study, and are a rich source of rebuses (see *Makaton National Curriculum Series. Part 1: Symbols*, 1993). As interest in rebuses and literacy has grown, simple word processing packages that include rebuses have been developed, for example *The Writing Set, Widgit*. The rebuses can be printed out and used in preparing games and materials.

Some features of early rebus systems are now viewed with caution and are not included in the current glossaries. Some of them made use of inappropriate semantic cues, such as a picture of a bee for the first syllable of 'began' or the picture of a knot to signify a negative. Picture cued words that combine picture symbol and printed word into one synthesized shape do still exist in current glossaries but are not recommended here. This practice has disadvantages; it may impair the view of the whole word shape, the visual processing of its constituent letters, and the formation of the automatic letter–sound links that we should be aiming to teach. It may also impede the understanding that, although text and pictures are linked, they are separate; we read the text, not the pictures.

It is the authors' experience that rebus symbols are a useful support to learners with specific difficulties in the areas of speech, language and literacy. They give extra support in making the link between the real object and its spoken and written form. Learners who have problems in storing the phonology of a word respond well to semantic cues, and a picture can enable recall. The single symbol for each word gives a semantic rather than a phonological cue, and makes no demands on sequencing ability. However, they must be used as part of a multisensory approach that has eyes, ears and hands firmly focused on an automatic response to print, or learners will pay too much attention to the rebuses and too little to the written words that accompany them.

The use of rebuses as an aid to literacy is not confined to special schools. As part of our work in supporting mainstream colleagues we have found teachers enthusiastic about introducing them into their practice.

Computers and Literacy Difficulties

The use of computers for learners with literacy difficulties is an exciting and rapidly developing area. Some dyslexic learners with good logical reasoning will have few problems in learning computer skills. Their ability to use and create computer programs can have good effects on self-esteem, as well as giving them a tool that facilitates written communication and encourages development of literacy skills. The explosion of multimedia packages onto the market for those with CD-ROM facilities is adding an exciting new dimension. The concept of literacy is changing as computer literacy becomes increasingly important.

Word Processing

Although there are many computer programs on the market aimed at improving the skills of dyslexics, it is word processing that currently offers the most exciting opportunities. Word processing allows the learner to write without inhibiting the flow, and to redraft and correct spellings later. As errors are easily and tidily corrected on the screen, it can give the confidence to attempt spellings that might not be attempted on paper. Once a first draft is completed, the writer can be encouraged to look for errors and to correct these straight onto the screen, or use the draft printout of the text to mark corrections needed before beginning editing. If a printout of the first draft is saved, it can become a record of progress and a pointer to where further help is needed.

For those learners with handwriting difficulties, the use of a word processor takes away the frustration and overload of remembering letter formation and joinings on top of correct spelling and language composition. It can dramatically increase the speed and quality of the writing as well as the motivation. It is important that the word processor should be used as a compositional and redrafting tool, not just as a means of typing out good copy.

Spell-checking devices built into word processing packages can point out spelling errors that a writer may have missed. Spell checkers may be used continuously as the writing is produced, or used afterwards to check through a text. Some recent devices such as *PAL* (Scretlander) offer a predictive facility where the computer tries to predict the words a writer is trying to spell, and gives spelling suggestions, as the writer types them. It builds up a personal dictionary for the user based on the user's own vocabulary and so is able to predict more accurately.

Talking Computers

The recent addition of speech synthesizers to word processing packages adds a whole new dimension, particularly those packages that offer immediate speech feedback (ISF). With this, parts of words, words and sentences can be read back to the writer by the computer. The quality of the sound is improving, and although it sounds 'robotic', the learner can hear as well as see what has been written. Hearing what has been written enables the writer to spot errors that an ordinary spell-checking device might miss. The learner also has the opportunity to change the spelling through listening to the speech of the computer. This requires rehearsal and further refinement of phonological processing skills and letter–sound correspondence. As a whole sentence is read back by the computer, syntactic errors that the writer has made may also be noticed.

It is an understatement to say that not all word processors are easy to use! For younger learners and for those with more significant problems there are simple programs such as Phases that allow for straightforward composition and basic editing of text. Some of the word processing packages currently on the market are too complicated for many of our learners, so care should be taken when making a choice. For an up-to-date guide to more recent developments, contact the British Dyslexia Association Computer Resource Group, 98 London Road, Reading RE1 5AU, UK, or the Dyslexia Computer Resource Centre at the University of Hull. Interested teachers might like to look at The Talking Computer Project (Miles and Clifford, 1994), and at the book by Singleton (1994) on computers and dyslexia (1994).

Concept Keyboards

A concept keyboard is an extension to an existing keyboard and is an extremely valuable resource. It opens up the use of the computers to younger learners and those with learning difficulties. It consists of a board divided into pressure points, which when pressed respond like the keys on the main computer keyboard. Overlays that correspond to the software being used on the computer are placed over the surface of the concept keyboard. The overlays are divided into areas that contain pictures, words or letters, which when pressed appear on the screen. A concept keyboard can be used instead of the main QWERTY keyboard, or alongside it. Overlays can easily be designed by a teacher without computer programming knowledge, and can be tailor-made to serve the needs of particular groups or individuals. Concept keyboards can be used to link in with a wide variety of computer programmes, from simple matching activities to adventure games. Many existing programmes already in use in schools can be accessed through concept keyboards.

The use of concept keyboards alongside simple word processing programmes opens up a wealth of opportunities. The overlay for the keyboard can be arranged alphabetically with lower case letters, and can include picture clues for those who need reminders of the sounds that the letters can make. These can be linked to the picture clues used in the reading pack described on p.101.Overlays can be made up of onsets and rimes to aid spelling. Whole words can be included, creating a word bank similar to those used in *Breakthrough to Literacy* (p.71). Overlays can consist of pictures or rebus symbols or can be a mixture of all these ideas. The list is endless, but the guiding principle is to provide the support that the developing reader and writer needs.

A recent development called *Clicker 2* (Crick Computing) enables a keyboard layout, similar to the concept keyboard overlay, to be incorporated onto part of a computer screen. Words or letters are selected through clicking on them with a cursor controlled by a mouse or another switch device. Individualized grids can be made and stored for future use.

Part 2:
Skills into Action

The 'Skills into Action' programme describes in detail an integrated approach to literacy skills. It begins with a chapter on assessment that provides an 'assessment menu' from which the reader can choose. This is then linked to the setting of learning objectives to include in Individual Educational Plans. 'Skills into Action' gives ideas for developing literacy skills through whole language approaches such as shared reading and writing. The chapter on phonological awareness includes practical ideas for developing awareness of rhythm, rhyme, alliteration, onset and rime, and phonemes, with suggestions for linking these with real reading and writing. A further chapter describes how to help learners improve alphabet and dictionary knowledge. A detailed, structured multisensory approach to letter sound correspondence follows, with guidance on planning lessons for individuals or groups.

Chapter 6:
Assessment

Part of normal classroom teaching practice is to assess the needs of the individual child across the whole spectrum of difficulties. The DFE Code of Practice (1994) describes a five-stage model of definition and assessment of Special Needs:

Code of Practice (DFE, 1994, p. 3).

Stage 1: class or subject teachers identify or register a child's special educational needs and, consulting the school's Special Educational Needs coordinator, take initial action.

Stage 2: the school's SEN coordinator takes lead responsibility for gathering information and for coordinating the child's special educational provision, working with the child's teachers to draw up an Individual Educational Programme (IEP).

Stage 3: teachers and the SEN coordinator are supported by specialists from outside the school in drawing up and implementing the IEP.

Stage 4: the LEA consider the need for statutory assessment and, if appropriate, make a multidisciplinary assessment.

Stage 5: the LEA consider the need for a statement of special educational needs and, if appropriate, make a statement and arrange, monitor and review provision. An IEP is usually drawn up in response to the statement and is regularly reviewed.

It is not until Stage 3 that the school is supported by specialists, including educational psychologists, from outside the school. At Stage 3, it may be necessary for the child to have a multidisciplinary assessment, perhaps calling upon an educational psychologist or a communication therapist. Before that, the teachers in the mainstream school need to be confident and knowledgeable about assessment, testing, drawing up IEPs, and in developing efficient teaching and learning routines. In setting up an IEP we should consider:

1.   what can the child do?
2.   what are the long-term objectives of the educational programme?
3.   what are the short-term objectives of the programme?
4.   what steps can the learner take?
5.   what support is needed?
6.   what approaches and resources are required?

Careful assessment is the first step. If the child has a Statement, it provides a basis for the Individual Educational Programme.

The Assessment Menu

The authors' emphasis is on an assessment of educational need, not on a diagnosis of what is 'wrong' with the child. We need to note what the child knows, but they can often have isolated bits of information that are not usable in the day-to-day tasks of thinking, reading and writing.

The first step in assessment has to be the assembly of a thorough, wide-ranging picture of the learner. Tests are only part of the picture; assessment takes place in the classroom and at home each time the child and adult interact.

Tests can be formal or informal. The model offered by the authors is by no means comprehensive; here are simply some tests and routines that have been found to be useful in devising suitable programmes for children with literacy difficulties. Not all the tests and routines will be necessary for all the children; the teacher will need to use judgment to select appropriate items from the menu.

Gathering Information

1.   Information from medical records about deficits in hearing or sight. Perhaps the child needs a new hearing or sight test. There may also be a record of earlier intervention from speech therapy services.
2.   Information from teacher (concerns, strengths, approaches used, books/schemes used, motivations, interests, samples of work).
3.   Information from pupil (interests, concerns, strengths, attitude).
4.   Information from parents (concerns, medical history, reading and writing at home, family literacy, willingness to be involved in the programme).
5.   Information from other professionals currently involved (e.g. speech therapist, educational psychologist).

Check Concepts About Print

1.   Does the child understand how spoken language is presented in a written form (orientation of book; print, not pictures, carries the message; direction of print; line sequence; page sequence; meaning of punctuation marks?

2.   Is the child familiar with the terminology used in reading instruction (front, back, word, letter, sentence, beginning, start, middle, next, end, page, full stop etc.)?

Marie Clay's Observation Survey (1993a) describes her *Sand* (1972) and *Stones* (1979), two little books that have been specially printed to give examples that test children's knowledge of these concepts. The Observation Survey gives instructions in their use, and normalized scores.

Check Phonological Awareness

1.   Awareness of rhyme.
2.   Production of rhyme.
3.   Awareness of alliteration.
4.   Production of alliteration.
5.   Copying rhythms.
6.   Counting syllables.
7.   Segmenting into onset and rime.
8.   Blending onset and rime.
9.   Segmenting into phonemes.
10.   Blending phonemes.

We have used a variety of resources for assessment of sound awareness. Lynette Bradley's (1980) *Assessing Reading Difficulties* provides detailed and simple diagnostic tests to identify problems with sound categorization, and suggests remedial procedures.

Peter Hatcher's (1994) *Sound Linkage* provides a rich source of materials to assess and improve the ability of a child to process sounds, and offers a programme that requires the child to integrate phonological skills with real reading and writing.

Gorrie and Parkinson's (1995) *Phonological Awareness Procedure* identifies difficulties and provides guidelines for their remediation. The procedure is divided into four stages: repetition of words and non-words, syllable segmentation, intrasyllable segmentation (onset and rime and rhyme), and phoneme segmentation.

Check Alphabet and Dictionary Skills

1.   Matching letters.
2.   Matching letter strings.
3.   Letter names.
4.   Alphabetical order.
5.   Writing alphabet.
6.   Writing individual letters to dictation.
7.   Dictionary skills.

Observing an older child write the alphabet can be the most instructive test of all—even if they feel that they 'know' the alphabet, you may observe that they have to repeatedly start at the beginning, and correct confusions as they go along. The Marie Clay Observation Survey (1993a) offers check sheets that can be used in testing knowledge of the above. Teachers can easily draw up their own.

Check Letter Sound Correspondences

1. Saying sounds of individual letters.
2. Writing letters to represent single sounds.
3. Saying sounds of consonant blends.
4. Writing consonant blends.

Keep a record of which letter sounds are known and use this later to see the progress the learner is making. The letter sheet included on p.124 can also be used as an initial assessment tool.

Check Word Recognition

1. Matching words.
2. High frequency words (see p.105).
3. Common irregular words.
4. Social sight vocabulary.
5. Keywords for school subjects.

Make a list of words known, and use this later to evaluate progress.

Check Strategies Used in Reading Aloud (Non-Standardized Tests)

Sometimes the child remains silent and waits for help, asks for help, or says that they don't know the next word. Such behaviour suggests an inactive approach to reading, and a lack of optimism about the chances of understanding or enjoying the book. In this case there is lots of work to be done in sharing the pleasure of books and stories, and finding simple and exciting stories and information that will motivate a reader. Self-correction, when a mistake that compromises meaning has been made, is a very positive sign; readers show that they are not merely 'barking at print'. If the child makes a substitution, it can be helpful to analyse the cues that the child is using, gaining insight into their strategies, so that strengths can be built upon, and ignored strategies can be introduced.

Marie Clay's (1993a) *Observation Survey* describes techniques in keeping a running record. They provide great insight into the strategies used by the learner.

In the *Reading Miscue Inventory Manual,* Goodman and Burke (1972) categorize the reader's substitutions in their miscues analysis.

Cliff Moon, in his (1990) article in *Child Education*, offers a simplified version of the Goodman and Burke miscues analysis that is easy to use. They suggest that the teacher should listen to the reader read a short passage (about 100 words) and note down any mistakes made. Do these errors show the reader is:

1.   Using visual cues: does the given word share at least half the letters of the target word, has the target word a similar shape (e.g. house, horse)?
2.   Using sound/symbol cues: does the child respond to the initial sound, to a letter cluster, to a syllable, to onset and rime?
3.   Using syntactic cues: does the substitute word have the same grammatical function as the target word (e.g. *is* for *was*)?
4.   Using semantic cues: does the given word have a similar meaning to the target word (e.g. *Daddy* for *Father*)?

Check Reading and Spelling Level (Standardized Tests)

The careful assessment you have made, like those used by Reading Recovery teams (Clay, 1993b), can tell you a lot about the strategies the child is using, and can indicate the useful elements of a remedial programme. Further information can be gained from the results of standardized tests. The important thing is to bear in mind the limitations of the test being used, to have a clear idea of the purpose of the test, and to use its result in conjunction with all the other information gathered. The reading age indicated will vary from one test to another. The reading age will tell us nothing about the strategies being used, neither will it indicate useful courses of action. It will not tell us anything about the strengths and weaknesses of the learner. Its indication of progress will be crude—learners who are improving some of the skills that underpin literacy may not make any progress on the test for months, and this can be very discouraging—and you may need something less crude. The authors test for two main reasons:

1.   It can be helpful to see how an individual compares to other readers of the same age. In a special school, a individual's ability can be misleading, and it is easy to underestimate the problems that could appear in a mainstream classroom. A test that tells you how a child's ability compares with others of the same age can give professionals and parents a realistic view of the possible difficulties to be overcome.
2.   A standardized test can be repeated to give an objective indication of the progress of an individual over a period of time. Parents have a right to such information, presented in a way that a layperson can understand. The tests described below are used by the authors, but there is no attempt to provide a balanced review; like most teachers, we use the tests available in the schools where we work. Tests are expensive, and have to compete for scarce resources with reading books.

Single Word Tests:

Schonell Graded Word Reading Test (Revised 1971) Oliver and Boyd.
Graded Word Reading Test; the Macmillan Test Unit NFER Nelson

Non-Word Reading Tests

Dyslexic learners have poorly developed skills in phonological decoding, and find it particularly difficult to process new words (see Rack, Snowling and Olsen, 1992 for a review). The *Graded Nonword Reading Test* (Snowling, Stothard and McLean, 1996) can tell the teacher if the learner's non-word reading score is at an age-appropriate level, and highlight any specific difficulty with decoding.

Sentence Reading

Suffolk Sentence Reading Test (Hagley, 1987) NFER Nelson is a multiple choice sentence completion test. It is simple to administer to individuals or groups, and covers reading ages 6 to 13.

Reading Text:

Individual Reading Analysis (Vincent and de la Mare, 1990). This measures comprehension and accuracy, converting the scores into age equivalents. It allows diagnostic analysis of reading strategies, on the lines of miscues analysis, and notes reading behaviour (age range 5;6 to 10 years.).

Neale Analysis of Reading Ability (Neale, British adaptation by Una Christophers and Chris Whetton, 1994) measures accuracy, comprehension and reading rate, and includes a diagnostic form for miscues analysis. The authors have a slight personal preference for the texts and pictures of the Individual Reading Analysis, but the Neale is extensively used, and measures children from 5–13 years of age.

Single Word Spelling Tests

Schonell Graded Word Spelling Test (Revised 1971, Schonell, F.J.). *Graded Word Spelling Test* (Vernon, 1977). Both these tests are very simple to give to individuals or groups, and the scores can be translated into an age equivalent, or spelling age (5years to 12+). You can gain good information about the child's strategies and needs from observing a learner taking these tests, especially if you look also at the free writing.

Check Free Writing

A look at the work done in the classroom can give a good indication of the child's approach and facility in written communication. To find out what strategies are available to the child, it is important to witness the act of writing. Emergent writers may only produce letter-like scribbles, but can indicate a knowledge that print conveys a message. A week later, the message can be forgotten, or changed. A child who is judged to have poor concentration in written work, or who is accused of using all sorts of evasive tactics to avoid getting on with the task, may have huge difficulties that ten minutes' observation can make clearly apparent. The difficulties may be due to:

1.   poor handwriting
2.   slow handwriting
3.   limited basic spelling vocabulary
4.   poor ability to 'invent' spellings
5.   poor ability to decide on salient points
6.   difficulties in thinking through a sentence
7.   a desire to express complex ideas with poor language skills

Save an annotated example of free writing that includes your observations and comments on the support the writer needed.

Spelling Analysis

Spelling in Context: Strategies for Teachers and Learners (Peters and Smith, 1993). A suitable passage of dictation is given (ages 5 to 14). The teacher is helped to identify the developmental stage reached, with guidance for the development of independent spelling strategies.

Assessment in Action: Two Examples

The assessments described below will give the reader an idea of the way teachers can move about the 'menu', picking out appropriate items, sharing information, and building up a picture of strengths, weaknesses, and educational needs.

1. Mark

Initial Observations

Mark moved into a new Y6 class in September. His teacher had taught his older sister, and was interested to find that Mark seemed to have a similar learning style, and similar problems. He found reading aloud embarrassing, and was very inaccurate. He could cope adequately with reading tasks within the classroom. His writing was poor, scanty, and badly spelled, though it was usually possible to understand it. In oral work, Mark was bright and responsive, and displayed a good general knowledge. Mark used common sense and imagination in practical tasks. He was quick to master use of the new class computer. He still had problems in learning his tables, but was good at Maths, and working at the same level as the brighter children in the class. The teacher felt confident in Mark's cognitive ability, and in his active and industrious approach to his work. She felt that his written work reflected neither his ability nor the efforts he made. She discussed Mark with the Special Needs Coordinator (Stage 1 of the Code of Practice), who said that Mark had had extra help with reading in Year 3, but had made good progress, and his Y4 and Y5 had not mentioned any problems. It was decided that the views of Mark's parents would be sought.

Gathering Information

In the fourth week of term the parents attended an open evening. The teacher mentioned her anxieties, and the parents were very relieved that their anxieties could now be acknowledged. Mark had been seen by his former teachers as a rather immature child, with poor concentration, and slightly below average intellect. His sister, who had gone through primary school with the same reputation, had responded well to special needs help offered at secondary school, and was now approaching GCSE as a successful, bright learner. Her difficulties with spelling were seen to be dyslexic in origin, and she would be granted exam concessions. The parents felt that Mark was showing signs of similar development to his sister, and were delighted at the thought of getting extra help for him before he moved to comprehensive school.

Mark's LEA had a team of support teachers who could be called in to give advice and help at Stage 3 of the Code of Practice. Because Mark had less than a year to go before transfer to secondary school, the school and the parents decided to bypass Stage 2, and call in a support teacher to assess Mark's needs and to help them plan an individual educational programme for him.

The support teacher gathered the information set out above, talked to Mark who he found could converse intelligently on many subjects, and did not need to set the agenda. The support teacher agreed that it was not necessary to ask for an Educational Psychologist to assess Mark's cognitive functioning. He went on to assess Mark's reading and spelling levels.

Formal Tests

They worked through the Individual Reading Analysis. It was noted that Mark was cooperative, and his perseverance was normal. His reading rate was slow. He made no attempts to sound out unfamiliar words; he would guess from the context, and substitute a word with a similar meaning. If he made an error that altered the meaning, he would go back and self-correct. His answers to the comprehension questions were brief and competent. His age equivalent for accuracy (middle point) was 8;9 years, and for comprehension it was 10;2 years.

Mark then went on to do the Daniels and Diack spelling test, a test of individual words. Mark spelled correctly all the simple regular words like 'mud' and 'beg'. He also managed words with consonant blends, like 'lost' and 'plan'. Every-day irregular words caused problems; 'so' was 'sow', 'for' was 'fure'. More difficult words were spelled phonically: 'women' was 'wimin', 'great' was 'grayt'. His score of 16 gave him a spelling age of 6;7 years.

The support teacher felt that the gap between potential and achievement was a significant one. Each term, a member of the support team gathered together a group of children with specific learning difficulties. They spent one day a week as a group in a small special school for children with communication difficulties, and were given two hours of individual tuition in their base schools. They focused on the development of literacy skills, using the multisensory structured learning tech-niques described in this volume. Mark, his parents and his teachers agreed that it might be an ideal solution to the problem of giving Mark urgently needed, inten-sive help, whilst keeping him in close contact with his own curriculum and friends. Mark was given a place in the Literacy Skills Group.

Assessment Through Teaching

The individual and small group teaching sessions gave opportunities for further assessment. Details of Mark's understanding, knowledge and skills were noted, and his educational programme adjusted to this information.

Alphabet Knowledge

Using the wooden letters (see p.90), Mark showed that he was familiar with alpha-betical order. He had some name/sound confusions: g/j, w/u/y, c/s.

Sound–Letter Correspondence

Although Mark 'knew' most of the sounds, he did not use them for reading, and used them reluctantly and inefficiently in inventing spellings. Thus his teacher started him off at the beginning of the structure (p.124), intending to build in a quick and automatic response to the letters. Mark quickly learned and used individual letter sounds, and began to respond to consonant blends in reading. He was unconfident and erratic in using 'r' and 'l' blends and long vowel sounds in invented spellings, so that although initial progress through the structure was swift, his teacher needed to linger as the sticking points were reached.

Sound Processing Skills

Mark could count syllables, and identify initial and final sounds. He could identify rhyme, and generate it. He had problems with the sounds within consonant blends, and found it difficult to identify the sounds in two syllable words—he could not identify and hold onto consonant sounds in two syllable words (e.g. the 'g' of magnet) when using a simple dictionary (see p.93).

Social Language Skills

Mark was a friendly and sociable child, and got on very well with adults. His approach to other children was friendly, but somewhat robust; he needed to have it explained to him that another 'naughty' child in the group was only 8, and had difficulties in expressing himself. From then on, Mark enjoyed being 'fatherly'. Sometimes his teasing seemed cruel, though Mark was horrified when this was discussed; he really didn't mean to hurt. Back in mainstream, Mark's growing confidence was expressing itself as naughtiness in music lessons, and 'rudeness' to the part-time music teacher. Mark's special school and mainstream teacher both treated these issues in the same way. Mark needed advice in sorting out these problems; he did not need to be seen as a problem child.

Reading Aloud

Mark's teacher heard him read each time they met (three times a week). Between their sessions, he preferred to read silently, but was prepared to ask for help if a word held up meaning. He did not want to read aloud to anyone at home or at school. At the start of each new book his teacher made a 'running record', ticking each correct word. At the end of the reading session, they would work together on the words Mark had found difficult, discussing appropriate techniques. If one in ten words was incorrect, she would encourage Mark to choose another one, or ask him if he would try it, and give up if it was too hard, or ask a parent to read alternate chapters.

Analysis of Free Writing

At the beginning of the term, Mark was slow and inefficient in expressing himself in writing. Task completion seemed to be his main aim; get the writing done with so that he could go onto something more interesting. This piece (figure 6.1) was a typical example of 20 minutes' work. He asked for help in spelling 'hamster', 'golf' and 'go karting'.

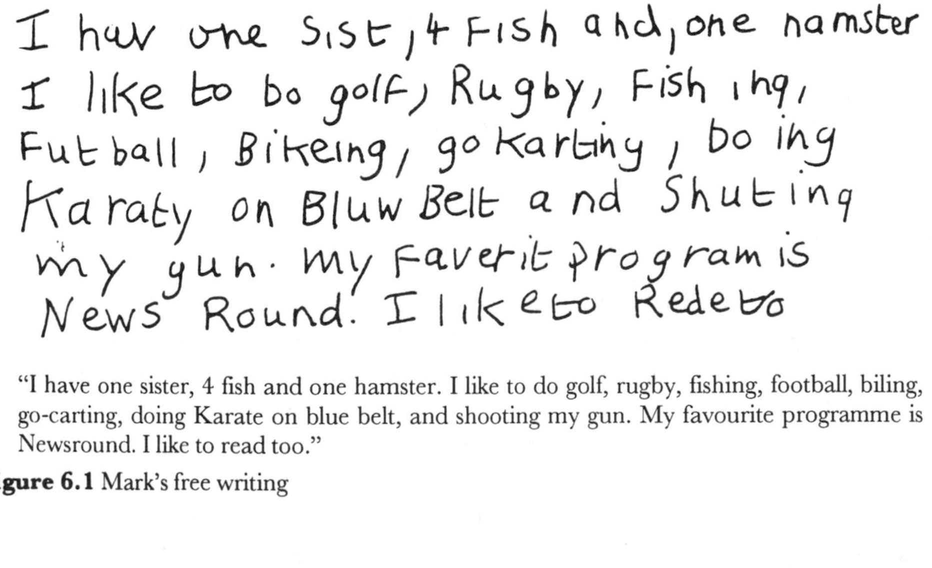

> I huv one Sist, 4 Fish and, one hamster
> I like to bo golf, Rugby, Fish ihg,
> Futball, Bikeing, go Karting, bo ihg
> Karaty on Bluw Belt a nd Shuting
> my gun. My Faverit program is
> News Round. I like to Redeto

"I have one sister, 4 fish and one hamster. I like to do golf, rugby, fishing, football, biling, go-carting, doing Karate on blue belt, and shooting my gun. My favourite programme is Newsround. I like to read too."

Figure 6.1 Mark's free writing

Using Frith's categories, Mark is seen to be using alphabetic techniques, 'sounding out' words like *faverit, futball*. He has some orthographic knowledge, and spells familiar words like *one* and *News Round* from memory. He seems to have some knowledge of rules, and adds a 'magic e' to lengthen the vowel sound in *Rede*. He knows that the /i/ sound at the end of words is usually spelled with the letter 'y' (karaty). His phonic knowledge is limited, and he seems to have developed no consistent way of spelling the oo sound (shuting/shooting, to/too). His handwriting suggests that he has attempted to eliminate b/d confusion by adopting the upper case form—though it is not always clear whether he is writing capital D with an extended first stroke, or lower case b (boing? Doing?). He uses commas and full stops correctly.

This sample of his work (figure 6.2), written eight weeks later, is again typical of the amount and quality of expression that he could achieve in twenty minutes:

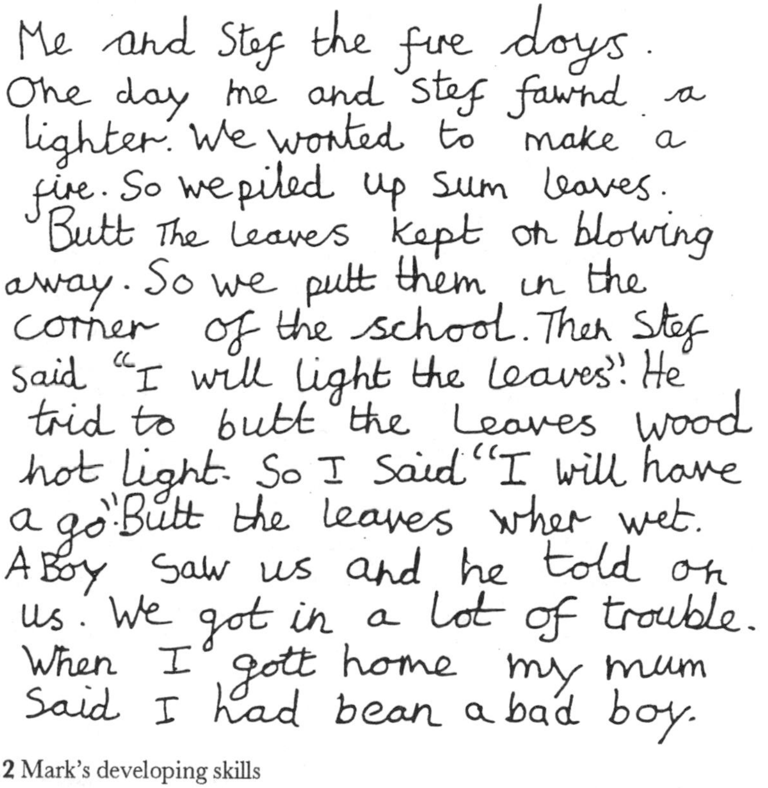

Me and Stef the fire doys.
One day me and Stef fawnd a
lighter. We wonted to make a
fire. So we piled up sum leaves.
Butt The leaves kept on blowing
away. So we putt them in the
corner of the school. Then Stef
said "I will light the leaves". He
trid to butt the Leaves wood
hot light. So I Said "I will have
a go". Butt the leaves wher wet.
A Boy saw us and he told on
us. We got in a lot of trouble.
When I gott home my mum
Said I had bean a bad boy.

Figure 6.2 Mark's developing skills

He looked up some words in a dictionary—'leaves' and 'trouble'. He asked for advice in spelling 'corner' ("is it cor-ner?"). His language is expressed in grammatical sentences, and he is beginning to mark them with correct pronunciation. He needs to know that a conjunction need not be preceded by a full stop, but he has mastered speech marks, and, except for 'Boy,' uses capitals correctly. His spelling mistakes do not hold up communication—'fawnd', 'wonted', 'wher', are good phonic attempts. He has noticed the generality that some cvc words double the final consonant (bell, miss, cliff), and over applied it to 'butt', 'putt' and 'gott'. These observations tell us where Mark has got to, and point us to the next things that need to be taught. However, the most exciting development is in the quality of expression—he has found his 'voice'. In personal relationships, Mark is kind, responsible, humorous and mature; he has found the confidence and skill to express this in his writing.

2. Jack

Jack arrived at a special school for pupils with moderate learning difficulties with a long history of language, literacy and behaviour problems. He had received additional support in one form or another for most of his school career, including language unit placement, but was still experiencing considerable difficulties in learning and literacy. Special school placement had eventually been sought and secured, after a long wait, during the first term of Year 9. Jack's teachers waited for the 'honeymoon period' to finish and for the behavioural problems to reappear; but they never really did. Perhaps at last he had the right level of support to meet his needs.

Gathering Information

Jack had been born full-term with a normal delivery. There had been no medical complications during his early childhood. His hearing, sight and physical development were normal. His social and emotional development had been delayed, and Jack had displayed frequent tantrums. He spoke phrases at 2 years, but his speech and language were delayed, and his speech was still unintelligible at 4 years. He received speech therapy and attended a language unit for 18 months. He was then transferred to a unit for pupils with moderate learning difficulties. At parental request he was transferred to a mainstream primary, and then moved on to secondary school. There, he received support for literacy, but had considerable difficulty in accessing the curriculum. His motivation and self-esteem began to suffer and his behaviour caused concern. His attendance was poor.

Over the years, Jack had received help in the form of *SRA Corrective Reading* (1988), and had used a range of reading schemes, including *Wellington Square, Fuzz Buzz* and *Oxford Reading Tree*.

Initial Observations

Jack appeared on the surface to be a student who was much more 'street-wise' than many of his special school peers, and it was initially feared that he might have resented the move. He was good at covering up the difficulties he experienced. However, the extent of his learning problems soon became clear. Along with his general learning difficulties, Jack had poor auditory discrimination. He had word-finding difficulties. He found it hard to remember the teaching he received. Psychological assessment showed that Jack had severe difficulties with working memory; because he could not easily process new information, he found it hard to learn and apply letter sound knowledge. Despite previous attempts at remediation of his literacy problems, he had made little progress. On arrival at his special school, he was still reading at the level of a 6-year-old. Despite his bravado and the image he was portraying to his peers, he cared very much about this, and wanted to improve the situation. Unlike Mark, Jack did not have other cognitive strengths to help him overcome his literacy problems; it was going to be a long haul.

Assessment of Literacy Skills

As Jack's reading was at such a low level, detailed formal standardized assessment was not considered to be appropriate. It was decided to take an inventory of literacy skills and knowledge that would form the basis of a future programme and a baseline for measuring progress. It would take some time before progress could be measured through reading age.

Reading

Jack read from his class reader, *King of the Road* (Nolan, 1976). He recognized a few words by sight. He attempted to 'sound out' unfamiliar words, but was unsuccessful. He made very little use of picture and context cues and needed to be reminded to do so. He did not appear to read for meaning; all effort was concentrated on decoding. There was no evidence of self-correction and he was unable to answer questions on the passage read.

Alphabet and Letter–Sound Knowledge

Jack had difficulty in reciting the second half of the alphabet, and was very slow in putting a set of wooden letters into alphabetical order. He frequently confused the orientation of the letters. Jack was able to give the correct letter sound for about three quarters of the alphabet. There were some name/sound confusions (k/q, b/d, y/j, i/e, u/n).

Word Recognition

Jack knew 26 of the 100 most common words. He scored a reading age of 6;7 on the Schonell graded word reading test.

Phonological Awareness

Jack was able to say if two words began with the same sound, and could give another word beginning with that sound. He was usually able to say if two words rhymed, but found it difficult to produce his own rhyming words. Following example, Jack could split words into onset and rime, and could blend onset and rime to produce words. With help, he could create new words through auditory analogy (e.g. given 'sip', and asked to change the first sound to /t/, could produce 'tip'). Jack could also count the right number of beats in one- to three-syllable words. He had particular difficulties in isolating, producing, and discriminating between vowel sounds. There were some immaturities in his speech (e.g. /f/ for /th/; difficulties in sequencing the sounds in multisyllabic words).

Writing

Jack was reluctant to spell words for himself. He relied heavily on a few keywords that he knew, and copied others from the teacher or from a dictionary. His diction-ary skills relied on first letter knowledge only. Jack's handwriting was usually a laboured print, but when asked, he could join some letters. There were frequent reversals and confusions over starting points.

It was decided that Jack would benefit from extra support for literacy even within the special school context. He became part of a group of four pupils in Year 9 who received additional literacy support three time a week. This consisted of two 40-minute group sessions, and an individual session of 20 minutes. For the rest of the week, Jack was taught as a part of his class group of 10 pupils.

An Assessment Summary

Keeping a single sheet that summarizes the assessment can be very useful for reference. Table 6.1 takes Jack's assessment as an example. Use this sheet to decide on learning objectives and to work out an Individual Education Plan (Table 6.2, p.60).

Continuous Assessment and Recording Progress

Keep ongoing records of progress made. Always include the date for newly acquired skills as rate of progress is equally important. Include regular annotated examples of the learner's free writing in your record keeping. These can be very informative for monitoring progress in the transfer of skills into a real writing context. Also include information gained from listening to the learner read. Note if the skills taught are being put into action by the learner in everyday reading. The diagnostic nature of our teaching programme facilitates continuous assess-ment. The step-by-step programme (p.119) provides a thorough diagnosis of the learner's knowledge and weaknesses in letter–sound links.

Table 6.1: Assessment summary		
Name *Jack*	D.O.B. *1.10.80*	Date *Sept. 1995*
Background information	*No medical difficulties. Behaviour poor in mainstream. Poor attendance. Low motivation and self-esteem. Parents supportive. Moderate learning difficulties.*	
Spoken language	*Delayed. Unintelligible at 4 years. Previously had speech therapy at language unit. Poor auditory discrimination. Word-finding difficulties.*	
Concepts about print	*Unsure of purpose of capital letters and full stops.*	
Phonological awareness	*Recognizes alliteration and rhyme. With example can blend and segment onset and rime. Can count up to three syllables. Difficulties discriminating between vowel sounds.*	
Alphabet and dictionary skills	*Difficulty reciting second half of alphabet. Slow in ordering the wooden letters. Confuses orientation of letters. Dictionary: first letter only.*	
Letter–sound correspondence	*Correct letter sounds most letters. Name/sound confusions $k/q, b/d, y/j, i/e, u/n$.*	
Word recognition	*Recognizes 26 of 100 common words.*	
Reading strategies	*Unsuccessful attempts at sounding out. Little use of picture and context clues. No self-correction. All efforts on decoding; none on meaning.*	
Standardized test results	*6.7 years Schonell Word Recognition test. Other tests not appropriate.*	
Handwriting	*Laboured print. Can join a few letters. Frequent reversals and confusion over starting points.*	
Spelling	*Wrote a few words from memory (the, and, is, it). Otherwise, copied from dictionary.*	
Free writing	*Refused to write without dictionary. Did not invent own spellings.*	

Table 6.2: Learning objectives *Literacy*

Name *Jack*	D.O.B. *1.10.80*	Date *Sept. 1995*

Concepts about print	*To understand the purpose of capital letters and full stops. To use these when writing a simple sentence.*
Phonological awareness	*To consolidate ability to blend and segment onset and rime. To use these skills when decoding or spelling simple three-letter words.*
Alphabet and dictionary skills	*To improve knowledge of letter names and alphabetical order.*
Letter–sound correspondence	*To reinforce initial letter–sound knowledge through use of a memory pack and through work on onset and rime.*
Word recognition	*To continue to build up sight vocabulary through shared reading and keywords in the structure.*
Reading strategies	*To encourage reading for meaning through shared reading and discussion. To encourage greater use of picture and context cues. To encourage use of onset and rime when decoding. Always relate back to meaning.*
Handwriting	*To improve letter formation and handwriting through a joined hand.*
Spelling	*To encourage the use of invented spelling through onset and rime*

Look ahead to p.115 to see how some of these learning objectives are implemented in a lesson plan.

Use a recording sheet (like the one on p.114) to keep track of skills teaching and learning. Compare the ongoing records you make with your initial assessment summary. This will help you plan for new learning objectives in your IEP. The lesson planning sheet on p.114 is linked to the assessment summary on p.59. It is also used to record difficulties or progress noted during a lesson and is used as a basis for further planning.

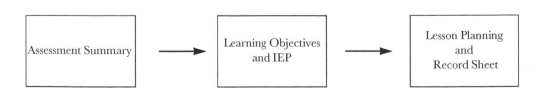

Figure 6.3 Moving from assessment to teaching

Chapter 7:
A Whole Language Approach to Reading and Writing

Shared Reading

As part of our approach to working with readers experiencing difficulties we would strongly advocate the use of shared reading (see p.33). It is through shared reading that we can stimulate a desire to read and create a link between the skills we teach and the use of these in real reading situations. We can encourage the development of the whole reader.

How might we use shared reading with learners experiencing difficulty? There are essential elements that we can adopt alongside our skills teaching. Some of them may seem obvious, but in our quest to overcome the specific difficulty many of our readers have, we can overlook these elements as we concentrate on isolated drills and routines. We need to ensure that skills are put into action. Shared reading can help us do this.

Listening to Stories

Read to the learners you work with. One of the problems for such readers is that, unlike successful readers, they do not experience enjoyment or learning through the medium of books. Perhaps we can compensate in some way for this by continuing to read to our slower readers and share books with them. Indeed, listening to someone read is a pleasure that we can all continue to enjoy, whatever our stage of reading development, as avid Radio 4 listeners will testify!

Introducing Books to the Reader

Introduce and become familiar with the books used in reading programmes before reading them (see p.33 for details of Holdaman's (1979) approach).

1. Discuss what the book might be about—look at the cover, pictures, title, publisher's blurb, etc. The same techniques are useful when choosing a book in a library or shop, and are part of the skills and anticipation of the enjoyment of reading.

2.   Make sure the book is not too hard for independent reading—try a simple 'running record', ticking each correct word (count self-corrections as correct). If one in ten words is wrong, or causing serious trouble, suggest that the book should be shared with a stronger reader.

Rereading Books

Creating a classroom culture of rereading books is an essential element of shared reading (p.33) . Try to avoid the response from learners, teachers and parents that once a book has been read it should not be attempted again. Rereading should be valued; it should be seen as support and not cheating. It has to be seen as a positive and pleasurable activity—we are not talking about the negative and dispiriting approach occasionally observed when a child has been 'put back' onto grade three from grade four because they don't know the words. There should be a common core of books that are accessible to the pupils and can be revisited many times. Activities that extend outwards from this core of books can be developed through games, drama, and the learner's own writing (see p.67).

Choosing the Texts

1.   Make sure they are appealing and relevant to the reader. We have used both 'real books' and reading scheme books according to the learner's needs. Home-made books and personal readers (p.63) can also be used.
2.   The language has to be meaningful and natural to aid prediction and understanding.
3.   A clear, easy-to-follow narrative style is essential.
4.   Stories that involve repetition and rhyme are useful. The structure is easily identified and draws attention to the similarities between words, letter strings and the sound of the language.
5.   Try poetry. Many modern children's poets (e.g. see Rosen, 1990) use simple words and short utterances to convey messages that appeal to learners whose mechanical skills lag behind their interests. Repetition has a purpose within the poem, rather than being a device to give the learner extra practice. They are also very funny, and learners enjoy preparing a poem and reading it aloud to their peers.
6.   'Big Books' are excellent for small groups and have now become a familiar part of infant school practice. They are larger versions of normal readers, and can be enjoyed by a group. Big books are available from many publishers, or can be home-made. Regular sized multiple copies of a book also allow groups to read together.
7.   Audio taped versions of stories allow revisiting of a text that a teacher or a group has shared.
8.   Not everyone likes fiction; use whatever is appropriate and motivating for the learner, including information books, computer games, magazines.

9.   Make personal readers. Home-made books can be centred around the interests and vocabulary of the individual pupils, and can overcome some of the difficulties of finding appropriate materials for children with impaired speech and language. Books can be produced that are at a level appropriate to individual development. The use of photographs of the pupils, or snaps they have taken themselves, can add to the appeal of such books. However, it is acknowledged that, no matter how well they are made, they can never take the place of 'real' books.

Use of Rebus

The use of rebus symbols (see p.37) can be a helpful prop to readers with literacy difficulties. Parents who have bought little activity books from the local post-office will be familiar with the idea—a picture is inserted into print, and replaces a word. This can introduce the toddler to the idea that a word is a unit, distinguishable from the flow of speech. The young child can 'read' with the parent, saying the illustrated words. Rebus symbols are pictures with print, but they are formalized, consistent images, and are used to accompany and illuminate a printed word. A rebus symbol can provide a key to a whole sentence, thus encouraging prediction and enabling the poor reader to gain valuable reading experience.

Some young learners need reading materials that are closely related to their own experience. Beginner readers can be made for them. For example, take photographs of the child, recording familiar activities, and use them for illustrations. Write a simple sentence beneath the picture, and add the rebus sign over each word. Provide cards with the rebuses and/or the words that can be used for matching games and activities. At this early stage of learning to read, rebuses on labels, timetables and instruction sheets can give independence to the beginner reader, encouraging the development of independent reading skills.

For older children (7+), the rebuses are more useful for the development of independent writing skills. The learner needs to have the ability to identify a letter that links the initial sound of a word, and to formulate and hold in short-term memory the sentence to be written. With this level of skills, words illustrated by rebus symbols can be kept in an alphabetical 'Word Bank' available to the whole class, or gradually collected in a personal word book (see p.72).

For struggling readers of any age, use of rebus symbols can usefully support activities used to help the learner increase sight vocabulary (see p.102). They can be added to a published story or to scheme books. Target a word that is causing immediate problems—with dyslexic learners, this is often a frequently used function word, where mistakes can encourage faulty prediction and throw out the rest of the sentence. Draw them above the text, using pencil, and rub them out when their support is no longer needed. They should not interfere with the scanning of the sentence—avoid the practice of interweaving the picture with the word.

Tom's use of Rebus

A description of a specific programme will provide an example and illustration of the use of rebus at different stages of reading development.

Tom's initial difficulties were in development of good language skills. He had significant word finding difficulties, and his pronunciation of many consonant sounds was unclear. He received regular speech therapy, and when he started school he had overcome the worst of his problems. Some remained—his pronunciation of consonant sounds was still 'fuzzy'. He pronounced /r/ as /w/, and /th/ as /d/ or /t/. He resorted to frequent use of 'thingy' and 'you know' when a word eluded him. In spite of these minor problems, he communicated well, and children and adults enjoyed conversations with him. He found it difficult to make a start on reading and writing. He loved listening to stories and enjoyed looking at books, and could invent plausible plot lines to go with the pictures. By the time Tom was approaching the age of 6, his teacher wanted him to focus on the words that were actually written. She maintained a full range of stimulating activities— Tom continued to enjoy sharing books, playing in the writing corner, and taking part in language groups; but she made him some personal readers. The first one charted his day at school. She photographed typical activities, and used the snaps to illustrate the book, writing a simple sentence under each picture, with the rebus sign above key words.

They read the book together, then played games, using cards with words and/or rebus symbols for matching games. Further similar books were made. Using photographs, or pictures cut from magazines, she made books on topics that interested Tom, using a limited vocabulary. As a word became part of his automatic sight vocabulary, its rebus sign was omitted.

Meanwhile Tom was starting a multisensory structured programme aimed at forming automatic letter–sound links. By the time he was 7, he could use the rebus symbols and his knowledge of initial sounds to access the Word Bank. He had a growing number of words in the alphabetic personal dictionary. He would try out a word he needed on a scrap of paper; if he spelled it incorrectly, and if he thought he might need that word again on another occasion, the teacher would print it into his dictionary, accompanied by its rebus.

At this stage, the use of rebus in reading development was limited to function words. For example, in one of his reading books the word 'with' appeared frequently. The initial letter was not much help to him–pronunciation of the /w/ sound was barely mastered, and didn't help much in establishing the phonic link. He was already familiar with the rebus (two simple interlocked ovals, like links of a chain). His teacher went through the whole book, drawing the symbol above the word 'with' each time it appeared. The word 'with' was also included in packs of more familiar rebuses and words used in various games. As Tom began to respond correctly to the word, support was gradually withdrawn, until he began to read the word without even noticing it. This approach was gradually extended to other important function words.

Using the Three Book Approach

The 'three book approach' can become part of the structure of our reading sessions. It includes one new book, one book that has been heard before, and one well known book. This is a real confidence boosting routine. With older learners, try using single pages or favourite sections of a longer book, poems or short stories. If there is not enough time for a three book approach, at least use two texts, one familiar and one new.

Reading Together

Encourage learners to read alongside you as you read. Reading alongside another reader is more supportive than reading *to* someone. As teachers, we have experienced the success of this approach with a range of learners with language difficulties, including dyslexia. It eases the pain of being unable read, to access or to pronounce all the words. It has even proved successful with those who are reluctant to communicate, and might be described as electively mute.

Listening to Reading

Use the *prepare–pause–prompt–praise* routine (Wheldall, Merrett and Colmar, 1987) when listening to the learner reading.

Prepare: once readers have a certain level of skill let them prepare for reading aloud. If we as skilled readers were asked to read aloud to someone, surely we would still want to rehearse our performance? Remember, reading aloud is a different skill from silent reading.

Pause: don't jump in too soon when the reader stumbles or hesitates; pause, giving time for skills to be put into action. After a pause of five seconds:

Prompt: say the correct word, and ask the reader to repeat it, or to repeat the whole sentence. If appropriate, suggest skills that might be used to decode the word.

Praise: remember to praise the reader when the word has been identified or self-corrected. Continue to praise throughout.

Exploration of Texts: Developing Skills and Strategies

Each reading session can be an opportunity to assess the techniques that the learner is using, and to encourage the development of skills and strategies appropriate to the task in hand. We are careful to announce that we are about to use a page or a section of the book for this purpose. If you have been providing an unobtrusive scaffolding, quietly murmuring the difficult words after a brief wait for the learner's independent efforts, it can be disconcerting if you withdraw the support without warning.

Encourage the Learner to Read for Meaning, Using Context

Say:
  Can you guess what that word might be?

Did that word make sense? Can you think of a better one?
Can you get a clue from the picture?
Read the whole sentence, then see if you can guess the hard word.

Encourage the Reader to Increase Sight Vocabulary

Scan a passage, looking for a specific problem word.
Copy a sentence, read it, and cut into individual words. Ask the learner to reassemble it. A more able learner will be able to do the same thing, omitting the reading stage, and 'test' the teacher.
Keep a list of target words you have worked on, and check them daily.

Encourage Letter–sound Analysis

Say:
That word made sense, but can you work out the right one? Look at the first letter.
You can work out that whole word (make sure that it is true! It might be necessary to divide the word into onset and rime).
You can divide that word into syllables.
Can you see any little words in that big one?

Draw Attention to the Strategies Being Used

Say:
That was a difficult word, well done! How did you work it out?
That's a new word, isn't it? How did you guess what it said?
You remembered that word from yesterday—well done!
Did you work that out from the picture? Well done!

Use the texts to create a direct link between specific skills teaching and real reading; this is an essential part of the development of integrated skills. Use the book you are enjoying together to illustrate the sound–letter links you are painstakingly reviewing. Once this way of working is established, the learners themselves might notice and point out similarities and differences in words. With the adult as a supportive guide, the learner can be encouraged to use a variety of strategies when reading, putting the Adams model of the reading process into action.

Developing Writing Skills

Encouraging Emergent Writers

The classroom climate, and the teacher's attitude towards writing, are crucial. We need to find ways to enable our learners to explore written language in the same way that browsing through the book corner or library, or sharing books, facilitates the development of reading. The adult's role as guide or scaffolder is similar to the one described for shared reading. The contexts for written exploration are as important as the contexts for spoken language and reading. Young writers are much more likely to pay attention to the quality of their message, to indistinct letter formation, and to self-correction of spelling errors when they feel a real purpose in getting their message across and understood (see Peters and Smith, 1993). We need to examine whether we as teachers always provide meaningful writing contexts for our young writers.

The Writing Corner

Establishing a writing table or corner that is permanently available is an ideal way of facilitating writing for learners of all ages, and at all stages of development. The corner should include a selection of:

papers and card of different size, shape and colour.
envelopes.
pencils, crayons, pens and markers.
scissors, rulers, hole punchers, staplers.
elastic bands, paper clips, paper fasteners, string fasteners.
clipboards and files.
plastic stencils.
pritt sticks, self-adhesive labels.

It should also include resources for supporting spelling such as word banks, diction-aries, and topic words. Examples of handwriting and different sorts of lettering should also be included for reference.

Add in additional surprises to ring the changes and to create new interest with office materials such as phones, directories, yellow pages, diaries, an old type-writer. Try school sundries such as registers, exercise books, timetables, black-board and chalk, shoppers' catalogues, newspapers, holiday brochures, postcards, greetings cards, shopping lists, menus, leaflets, old forms, library tickets etc. These items can spark off new reasons for writing, and discussions about print. How these are used will depend on the age and maturity of the child. The inclusion of a message board or post box in the writing corner will allow the development of all sorts of written dialogues between learners, staff and visitors.

The writing table needs to be established alongside a culture of writing for a purpose, and of drawing the attention of the learner to print in the environment. The adults and other children in the class act as models demonstrating the communicative nature of print and as recipients of, and respondents to the writing attempts. This can be done formally through adult and learner writing together to create a caption to accompany a drawing, a model or an event in the learner's day. It can also be done informally, by learners exploring the writing corner for them-selves.

Book Making

Making books in the writing corner in response to books that have been shared is an excellent way of increasing the learner's understanding of written language and their writing skill. Younger pupils will often do this spontaneously. Some may prefer to respond to books they have enjoyed by writing a book review that can be displayed on the message board.

Older learners with literacy difficulties can also enjoy making books for themselves or for younger children. We have been involved in successful projects where older pupils made books for younger ones. They had to find out what the younger children liked, and what style and complexity of books they were able to read. This activity proved to be an enjoyable and age-appropriate way of encouraging older learners to write simple sentences, using relevant keywords. It is only through writing that we come to understand what sentences are, as we often do not use complete sentences in our spoken language (see Whitehead, 1990). The 'research' also gives older learners a legitimate reason for reading books that are simple and enjoyable, but might otherwise be seen as 'babyish'. Making books can allow some learners with poor literacy skills to shine by using good artistic talents. *A Book of One's Own* by Paul Johnson (1990) contains a wealth of ideas for making books with imaginative formats, and ideas for stimulating discussion about stories.

Letters

Letter writing, both inside and outside the classroom, provides an exciting context for writing. It can be encouraged in the writing corner. It can include writing to another class or school, perhaps creating a link with another town or country. Try writing to members of the local community who have been involved with the learners. Children of all ages love receiving mail, which spurs them on to write some more!

Talk to the parents, and encourage the learners to write to members of the family. It can be overwhelmingly pleasing when a learner with delayed literacy development first writes a note to the family (two scribbled notes, "Jeen wrang will call agen" , "Gon to shops back in a minit", were shown to us with tears of joy and pride!). It is a real mark of progress when the learner begins to use the new joined handwriting to thank Grandma for the Christmas present.

Newspapers

A class or school newspaper is an excellent way of developing the concept of the writing corner for older pupils. The corner can be set up like a newspaper office and production line where articles can be researched, written, edited, illustrated, etc. The use of a computer programme that enables the finished product to be realistic adds excitement to the venture and a sense of professionalism to the writers. Newspapers produced can be circulated through the school to friends, parents, governors, etc.

Links with Skills Training

The thoughtful teacher will be able to create links between the work of the writing corner and the skills teaching on phonics and spelling. Creating rhyming stories, riddles or poems enables the older child to practise writing words through manipulating onsets and rimes that may have been part of a formal spelling lesson. Use of these skills puts them into a meaningful context. The teacher will also be able to use observations made in the writing corner to decide what activities need to be included in a learner's structured spelling programme.

Invented Spelling

Once some letter–sound correspondence is established, the learner should be encouraged to use this knowledge to create spellings of words when writing. Creating a climate where invented spellings will be attempted is an extremely important part of the teacher's role in helping learners move through the emergent stage of writing into the alphabetic stage of literacy development. It is through the transfer of speech sounds to paper that the learner masters the alphabetic code both for reading and writing.

Invented spellings need to be encouraged from the start so that learners are willing to explore spelling for themselves, making use of more formal teaching of the letter sounds. The learners gain experience of using their growing knowledge and skills in sound blending. They also find unexpected ability to express themselves. Have a look at these two examples of Andy's writing (figures 7.1 and 7.2), done three months apart:

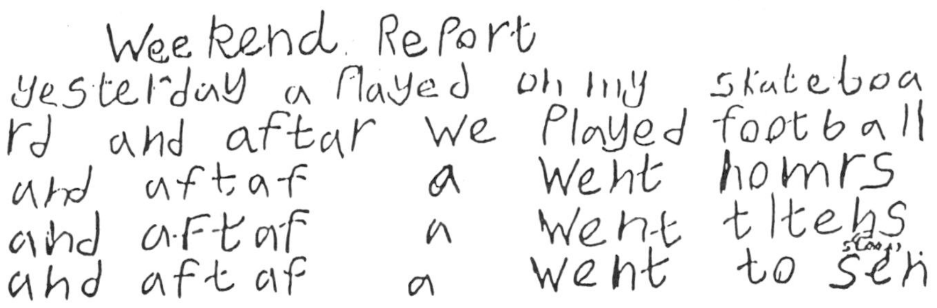

'Weekend Report: Yesterday I played on my skateboard and after we played football and after I went home and after I watched television and after I went to sleep.'

Figure 7.1 Andy's writing

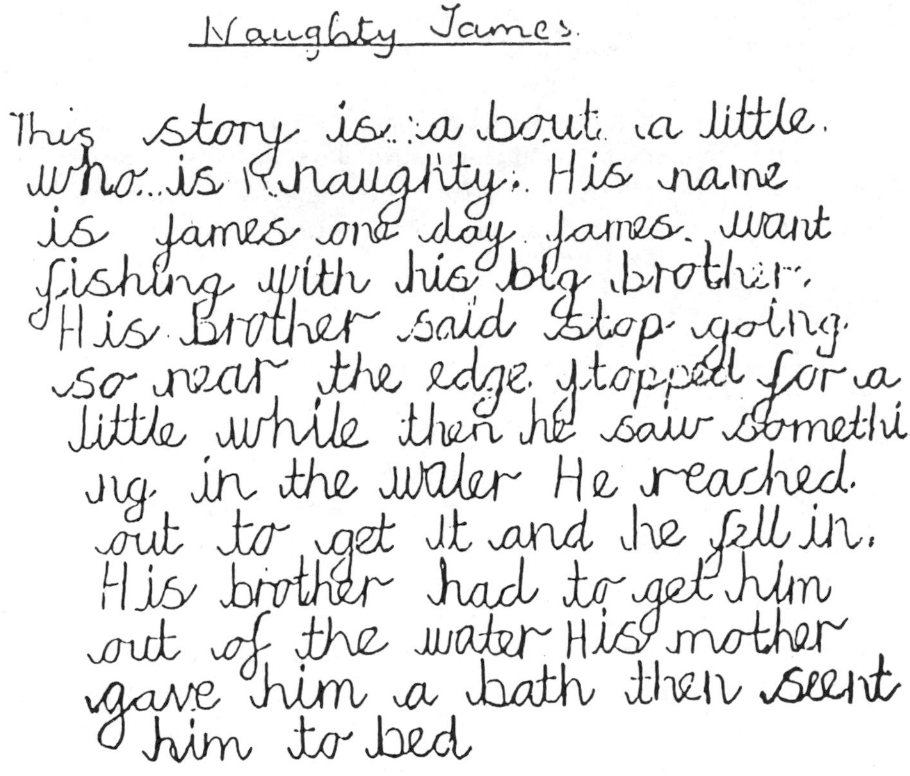

<u>Naughty James.</u>

This story is about a little.
who is naughty. His name
is James one day James want
fishing with his big brother.
His Brother said Stop going
so near the edge. stopped for a
little while then he saw somethi
ng. in the water He reached.
out to get it and he fell in.
His brother had to get him
out of the water His mother
gave him a bath then seent
him to bed

Figure 7.2 Andy's developing skills

The second example reveals an undoubted improvement in the skills of handwriting and spelling, and needs no translation. But the most striking difference is the freedom of expression—no longer does he have to rely on a small vocabulary of words he knows (or thinks he knows!). This freedom of expression is not an inevitable discovery, sometimes the ability to freely invent credible phonic attempts shows that the writer cannot decide what to put, and how to express it. The problem might be lack of confidence, but it may be the result of deeper language problems, where the learner has a limited ability to organize language into sentences.

Older learners who have not been brought up in a climate that allows spelling 'mistakes' may be reluctant to invent their own words, and may rely heavily on copying words rather than attempting to spell them. It is important that the teacher does not dismiss or over-correct the mistakes that are made. Playing with nonsense words and rhymes is one way of developing this skill in older learners—there is no 'right' answer to be anxious about.

Shared spelling is a supportive way of working. The teacher and learner can write a word together. The learner might write the letters for the first and last sounds, and the teacher can write the vowel sound between. The learner can overcome reluctance or inability to attempt a word by leaving a 'magic line' to be filled in later (e.g. 'ch___r' for chair).

'Best guess days' can be established. Learners are encouraged to have a guess at the spellings rather than automatically looking them up. As the learner progresses, best guesses and invented spellings can be checked later and corrected, but the teacher will have to use skill, restraint and diplomacy if they want to keep an atmosphere where the learner will 'have a go'.

Teacher as 'scribe'. In most infant classrooms you will see a young child dictating a sentence as a caption for a picture. A development of this technique also works well for the older learner. Many teachers and parents will feel that the dyslexic learner has a wealth of ideas and information, a good vocabulary, and a lively imagination. These are not expressed in writing because of difficulties with spelling or handwriting. However, taking away these pressures by using teacher as a scribe can reveal that there are also problems in organizing these ideas, deciding how to express them, and selecting appropriate detail. The teachers acting as scribes can find they are at the receiving end of a rambling, diffuse narrative almost as long as *War and Peace*. Alternatively, they can be given a twenty-word summary of a story. Simple routines can provide a structure for the task:

1. Ask what the story is going to be about. The summary provides a structure to restrain and support the long-winded ones, and signifies to the terse writers that the actual telling of the story demands a different mind-set.
2. Decide who the story is for.
3. Ask the writer to define and name the characters.
4. Ask the writer to decide where the story begins (e.g. Joe got up? Joe had his breakfast? Joe went to the park? Joe was in playing in the park when suddenly.....?).
5. Ask the writer to decide on an ending. This helps prevent a never ending tale that rambles on and on, finishing only at the end of the page or when the writer has had enough.
6. Allow the writer to read the first draft through, and make changes—not just correcting minor errors, but making conscious literary decisions. Use a thesaurus to vary vocabulary. Use punctuation to add emphasis.
7. Discuss presentation. If using a word processor, allow the writer to play about with fonts and letter sizes. If the text is going to be made into a book, decide how big the chunks of text will be.

'Breakthrough to Literacy'

The 'Breakthrough' materials used in many infant classrooms (Mackay, Thompson and Schaub, 1978) work very well with older learners with writing difficulties. They are designed to allow the writer to concentrate on sentence composition, free from some of the anxieties of achieving correct spelling and handwriting. Pupils have a personal store of words printed on cards stored in a word bank called a sentence maker. They then use these words to compose sentences on a stand before writing them down. Letters can also be included for invented spellings. Punctuation marks are written on their own cards. Blank cards signifying and exaggerating spaces between words can be useful for writers who run their words together. Teachers and learners can discuss the language used and revise it before it is finally written down. New words can be added to the sentence maker as appropriate.

Personal Word Books

Personal word books can be a great support to some learners. Unlike published dictionaries, they accommodate the vocabulary and interests of the learner. They are much simpler to use if correct spelling is the purpose of the dictionary. They can have the added support of initial sound picture clues that can be linked to the clues presented on the reading pack cards (see p.101). However there is a tendency to over rely on word books at the expense of inventing and learning spellings independently. Once the learner has established letter–sound correspondence, word books should be used more sparingly alongside best guess days, magic lines and shared spelling. Their most important use is for checking spellings after they have been attempted.

The Concept Keyboard

The developing writer will benefit from overlays that might include whole words, letter sounds, rebus symbols or other picture clues. Personal wordbanks of keywords or topic words can be made for basic writing programmes such as 'Phases' (SEMERC). The developing writer presses the required word or letter sound on the concept keyboard overlay, and it appears on the computer screen. The writer can compose a text using whole words or a combination of words, letter sounds and punctuation marks. The inclusion of letter sounds allows the writer to use invented spellings (p.69) as part of the writing process. If necessary, the letters can be linked to the picture clues that are part of our structure (p.), giving added support. The finished piece of work can be discussed with the teacher, checked and redrafted, then printed.

The advantages of *Clicker 2* (see p.42) that produces the equivalent of a concept keyboard on the computer screen without the need for a separate device are obvious. However, learners with motor control difficulties might still benefit from the use of the concept keyboard.

Planning Stories

Very few writers produce a piece of work without some form of planning, review and redrafting. This aspect of writing is an important part of the National

English Curriculum. The use of a planner helps to structure the initial stages of the writing process. Burtis et al. (1983) suggest that the most effective planners are those that use visual forms such as flow charts or brainstorm webs rather than sentences or paragraphs. However, dyslexic learners often find it difficult to use a planner. If it is too complicated, many of them will merely copy the words or phrases on the web. It may be necessary to establish an understanding of the drafting process by acting as scribe whilst the learner uses the chosen plan to dictate the story. You may find you have to be quite prescriptive, asking for one whole sentence about each point.

Drawing Pictures

It is common practice to illustrate a story after it is written. Drawing the picture first can encourage a learner to start writing. The teacher can discuss the picture with the writer, drawing out the narrative (what is this person called? what happens next?). Write down keywords, discuss them and note special features about their spelling. This will help writers who rely heavily on a small, familiar, written vocabulary.

The successful use of pictures as a precursor to writing does depend on the willingness of the learner to draw. Younger children are less inhibited, but some older learners have the same doubts about themselves as artists as they have about themselves as writers. They need convincing that great works of art are not required. Once through this barrier, most writers find that preliminary drafting of their ideas in picture form is an excellent way of proceeding.

Picture Planners

The use of drawing can lead to the use of more structured picture planners. They can be used with learners at all stages of development. Most learners are familar with the cartoon sequences of comics and can enjoy planning out stories in a similar style. Keywords, written notes or dialogue can be added onto the planner and incorporated into the full version of the story written later.

First Draft

The learner should not worry too much about correct spelling and presentation at this stage. Writers who can invent plausible phonic spellings can be encouraged to concentrate on expression, putting marks against spellings that will need to be checked later. These spellings will be checked by the learner's own resources (personal word books, dictionaries) or with the teacher.

Redrafting

Using a word processor makes redrafting a relatively painless process (see p.40).

The text is easier to read, mistakes are easier to spot and to correct, and printing off drafts is easy. When a word processor is being used (which, with limited resources, usually means when it is the learner's turn) it is possible to achieve a higher standard of proof reading, and second, third or fourth drafts can be printed off. If the work is being done by hand, second drafts are usually final drafts, except for very special efforts.

Proof Reading

1.   Ask the writer to read through the text, putting a mark against any mistake they find. (see Peters and Smith,1993, *Spelling in Context: Strategies for Teachers and Learners* for ideas—they suggest a secretarial code for this process).
2.   Remind the writer to check for 'targets' that are currently the learner's responsibility (e.g. b/d reversals, spelling 'said' and 'they' correctly).
3.   Link with skills teaching—draw out relevant errors and discuss.
4.   Ensure that the writer has a manageable text to work from—correct any remaining mistakes, and discuss production of a second draft.

Evaluation

Once the final draft has been handwritten or printed, the work should be evaluated and celebrated.

1.   Teacher and learner comment on the piece of writing. What did the teacher admire or enjoy? What is the learner particularly proud of? How does it compare with their other pieces of work? Could the work be improved? What are the targets for the future?
2.   Share with others. Writer reads the work to peers, or to younger audience (some will need the teacher to read it for them—but only with permission!). Ask the listeners to make one positive comment each ('I liked the bit where......'; 'that bit made me laugh'; 'the drawings are really good'). Praise from peers, even within this formal setting, has wonderful effects on self-esteem, and helps to establish a group culture of joint support.

Rebuses and Writing

We stress throughout the book the importance of linking reading and writing through a multisensory approach. Rebus approaches that include the writing of words associated with the symbols will ensure that attention is given to the individual letters, their shapes, sounds and sequences, and not just to the symbols themselves. With this constraint, the use of rebuses can enhance the existing approaches to writing:

1. Draw the symbols on cards for the 'Breakthrough' word folders and sentence makers (see p.72) The symbols give additional support for new words that are being learned, or for those occurring as part of a class topic. In this way a greater variety of sentences can be produced and a greater sense of independence achieved.
2. Incorporate rebus symbols into wordbanks created through the use of concept keyboard overlays for computers (see p.41).
3. Include rebus symbols in individual word books, 'Breakthrough' word-banks, or personal dictionaries. The rebus can help the learner find the required word.

Punctuation

Writers can communicate well enough using alphabetic spelling skills—correct spelling is a nicety that can be developed over time, or corrected by computers or a proof reader. Much of the time, punctuation can be judged to be correct or incorrect. However, its use can obscure or convey the writer's meaning— it is an important part of communication. In conversation, we can use tone of voice and body language as well as words. In writing, we use instead typographical signs, colour and layout. Learning how punctuation works aids self-expression, and can be approached as an art rather than as a skill.

1. In shared reading sessions, draw attention to typographic signs. Point out that the listener will understand the passage better if the reader stops at full stops, and pauses at commas. Notice how the printer uses bold type or italics to emphasize certain words. Look out for exclamation marks and question marks, and use them to affect the reading. Explore together the graphics in comics.
2. Encourage the writer to use graphic print. It is fun to do ghostly letters for a ghost story, or to draw an exploding star round the word BANG! As the writer develops, explore together different forms of communication; comic-style graphics are not appropriate in formal communications.
3. Teach first the cruder and more obvious punctuation marks. Learners enjoy using exclamation marks, and their purpose can be easily understood. It is also very easy to see the purpose of a question mark. Make sure that the learner can 'draw' the mark properly—look at the different versions in various fonts, and make sure that they are written in the right zones. Notice that question marks and exclamation marks contain a full stop, and have the same grammatical function.
4. Before using speech marks, make picture stories with 'speech balloons' that contain the words the characters are saying. Older learners enjoy adding dialogue to photographs cut from magazine ads—especially the love scenes! Point out that the speech marks work in exactly the same way; they only contain the words actually spoken. Notice the convention in comics for

putting a cloudy bubble round words that are thought or subvocalized. Putting speech marks into a story written by the learner can be a useful part of redrafting.

5. Full stops can be introduced in skills sessions (see Sentence Writing, p.110). If young writers are encouraged to think out a whole utterance before writing, and to say it or subvocalize it, these utterances are very often rounded, grammatically complete sentences. Adding stops to mark these sentences is a part of redrafting. In time, and with encouragement, they become automatic at first draft stage.

6. Commas are tricky! They are most obviously useful in lists, but can also be introduced at the redrafting stage when phrases or clauses in a complicated sentence need separating to aid meaning.

7. Apostrophes are confusing, and often used wrongly to indicate plurals (Jean's, only £10.99! Apple's, 49p a pound!). They are important at an early stage in reading. The safest advice in the early stages is only to use an apostrophe to mark an omission–the **o** of **not** in **can't**, the **i** of **is** in **it's**. Teach possessive **'s** (Pat's coat, John's book) separately from contractions. The best advice about using apostrophes for writing is: If in doubt, leave it out!

8. Older learners might wish to communicate meanings that are complex enough to warrant use of colons or semi-colons. They could be introduced at the redrafting stage, but only by a teacher who is fully confident of their usefulness. They always separate main clauses that could be complete sentences. A semi-colon balances two statements of equal importance; a colon indicates that the second clause will elucidate the first.

Chapter 8: Developing Phonological Awareness

Improving the level of skills in this area is a slow business. As with the acquisition of knowledge of letter names and alphabetical order, there is no cut-and-dried sequence of activities, and the suitability of each one depends on the age, interests and stage of development of each learner. Some of this work will have been done before school. The pace of learning will vary according to the severity of the learning difficulty. The child with a deprived language background, but with a sound multisensory learning system, will probably progress more rapidly than the dyslexic child who may have received training, but needs very much more over-learning. Children with language development difficulties will need to have a programme developed in collaboration with a communication therapist, especially if they are currently working on awareness and pronunciation of certain speech sounds. The learner nccds to have some sound awareness before moving to the literacy programme, where the sounds are represented by letters; but it will be necessary to continue the oral work long after the written programme has been started. (Look back at Lahey's language model, p.5 to remind yourself of the inter-active nature of all language/literacy processes).

Developing a Sense of Rhythm

Circle games that involve copying or passing round a rhythm can be fun and many variations can be developed by both teachers and learners.

The leader starts a beat that is then tapped or clapped by the rest of the group seated in a circle (e.g. two short claps and one long one; one clap, two knee pats, two stamps of the feet). The rhythm can be copied by all the group at once, or passed round individually until back to the leader who chooses someone else to start the next rhythm. The game can be made more exciting by changing the direction of the rhythm passed along by eye contact or by calling the name of a group member.

Use *percussion instruments* to carry the beat round the circle, or to accompany music. Remember some learners will find it more difficult to maintain a beat with an instrument; make sure they have the feel of the beat before introducing instru-ments—tapping is the easiest, then clapping. More accomplished learners can develop their own rhythms and compose short pieces to play to the rest of the group. Using unusual instruments such as household or classroom objects can add to the fun. Choose pieces of music with a clear beat, and vary the style of music according to the interests and age of the learners.

Play *'Band Leader'*. Circle members have different instruments or sound makers. The learners take it in turn to be band leader, conducting the 'orchestra' with a baton, setting the beat, and bringing in the players individually or in groups.

Use *visual clues* during rhythm activities. They give added support to those who have difficulty in remembering a sequence. A simple score sheet can be developed through the use of symbols to indicate the rhythm—dots can indicate short beats, dashes can indicate long ones. Strips of card can be used in a similar way—squares for short, rectangles for long. The learners can develop their own scores that can remind them of the rhythms they have created, and can be given to others to play.

Use the *whole body* to express a beat. This can be very difficult. It may be necessary for a learner to build up expertise by moving across the floor in simple rhythms (e.g. two steps, one jump, two steps, one jump) before attempting to move or dance in time to a beat or a piece of music. Visual clues can also support movement activities. Hoops can be arranged in different patterns, perhaps with number or picture clues inside, indicating the number of hops, steps, jumps, etc. that make up the rhythm. Many simple folk or country dances can be used to develop a sense of rhythm. For the older and more cynical, try aerobic exercise or disco dancing. Even the Mr Motivator video has been used successfully!

Rhythm Within Spoken Language

Awareness of syllables springs naturally from the activities already described. The following activities will help to make the links explicit. Be aware that the word *syllable* will probably be unfamiliar to the learner—explain that a syllable is a beat, and use the activities to help the learner to master the new vocabulary as well as the phonological skill.

Instructions can be given through rhythm by tapping or clapping the syllables, e.g. 'Please fetch the book' (4 syllables), 'Stand by the window' (5 syllables). Vary the emphasis made on different words by clapping the long and short beats: — .. — (Please fetch the book). Alternatively, the learner can use the blackboard to mark one dash for each syllable, and add an accent mark (/) over the word you choose to accent: '*Please* get my bag' , 'Please get *my* bag', 'Please get my *bag* '.

Choral recitations of poems and rhymes can be great fun and help to develop a sense of rhythm in the spoken word. Well-known nursery rhymes can be used with younger learners. Older ones prefer limericks, advertising jingles and short humorous poems. Learners can work in pairs to develop their own presentations, speaking lines simultaneously or alternately. Divide bigger groups into choruses speaking alternately from two sides of the room. Simple raps, appealing to older learners, can be performed in this way. Encourage discussion about the rhythm and syllables.

Play *chanting games*. 'The Cookie Jar' is a favourite. Say the words very rhythmi-
cally; sit in a circle, and alternately clap and slap the thighs to mark each syllable.

All: Who stole the cookie from the cookie jar?
Leader: (Chooses a name, e.g. Jane) stole the cookies from the cookie jar.
Jane: Who, me?
All: Yes, you!
Jane: Couldn't be!
All: Then who stole the cookies from the cookie jar?
Jane: (Chooses e.g. Owen) Owen stole the cookies from the cookie jar.........

Play *clapping games*. A favourite is played in pairs. The players clap their hands
together, then clap each other's hands. The pattern can be made more complicated (e.g. together, right, together, left, together, both). Say a simple rhyme in
time with the claps. A well known example is: 'A sailor went to sea, sea, sea; to see
what he could see, see, see; but all that he could see, see, see; was the bottom of the
deep blue sea, sea, sea...'. Older Primary school children can usually provide
further examples. It is a very good and amusing way of emphasizing syllables
within words, but may be too difficult for some.

Simple blending games can be played. The teacher speaks two or more syllables in
the correct sequence, and the learner has to blend them to find the mystery word
(e.g. ta-ble, al-pha-bet).

Segmentation games can be played in a similar way—say a word that has to be
spoken in separate syllables by the learner.

Syllable manipulation games are difficult, but fun—the learner has to manipulate
or delete syllables, for example: 'What's left if you take 'car' off 'carpet'? What's
left if you take 'net' off 'magnet'?' The Topsy Turvy game is harder: 'Switch the
syllables so that 'carpet' becomes 'petcar', 'jigsaw' becomes 'sawjig''.

The last three activities can be linked to board games—when the learner lands
on certain squares of the grid, a syllable task has to be completed before an extra
turn is won or a move can be made.

Use the learners' *names*. Demonstrate, clapping vigorously: "How many syllables? SI-MON. How many syllables? DA-VID. How many syllables? SA-MAN-
THA". The learner can tap or clap the syllables, or count them on the fingers. You
can move on to car names, or football teams, or television programmes. When the
learners have mastered the skill, let them take over the naming and clapping.

Linking Rhythm and Syllables to Reading and Writing

Once the learner has experienced some of the above activities, they should be
directly related to reading and writing. Remind the learner that each syllable
contains a vowel; the vowels are a, e, i, o and u (sometimes y).

Use *poems and rhymes* as texts for reading. Give the learners printed versions of
the rhymes they are using for recitations or choral speaking. The texts can be

marked by teacher or learner to show who is speaking, and which rhythm is to be used.

Use *shared reading activities*. Talk about the rhythm, and tap out the syllables of some of the words. This will aid pronunciation of difficult words (e.g. hippopotamus). Write the selected word out, and identify the syllable boundaries by marking them with a pencil. Notice that each syllable has a vowel. During independent reading of unfamiliar words, encourage the learner to identify the number of syllables and their boundaries, and to decode syllable by syllable (e.g. fan-tas-tic). (See section on onset and rime, p.84, for help in decoding syllables.)

Physically cut or split words into syllables to be sounded out and read (link also with onset and rime, p.80) Print the words to be split on cards or make them out of plastic or wooden letters. Make a set of jigsaws of two or three syllable words, a syllable on each piece of the jigsaw.

Spelling multisyllabic words is difficult. Take it in stages: tap out and count the number of beats, say each syllable separately, then write them out one at a time.

Play the syllable blending, segmentation and manipulation games already mentioned using plastic or wooden letters, or words written on cards. Board games could use printed cards to give the learner written instructions.

Developing Awareness of Rhyme

Explaining rhyme is not always easy. Rather than asking "Do these words rhyme?", let the learner first experience rhymes in action. Encourage the learner to listen to the end 'chunks' of words to hear if they sound the same.

Enjoy the pleasures of *rhymes and poetry* together. Read them aloud. Tape record them for further use—they can be enjoyed individually through headphones. Encourage discussion of poems, and make anthologies of favourites. Use poems and rhymes for texts in shared reading. Make sure there are good examples, appealing to your learners, in your book corner or library. Encourage the learning of short rhymes to recite. Notice (and appreciate) poems that do not use rhyme.

Reread familiar poems, missing out the rhyming words, encouraging the listener to say them. Try supplying alternatives to the rhymes chosen by the poet. Changing traditional rhymes is fun—pairs can work together on this and recite them to an audience.

Create oral poetry. Once learners begin to develop a sense of rhyme, encourage them to make up their own poems. Concentrate on the appreciation of sound similarities. Limericks are popular with older learners. Try devising rhyming advertising slogans.

Rhyming tag can be played in P.E. The person tagged can release themselves if they identify a word that rhymes with one given by person who has tagged them.

Rhyming chain is a simple circle game where each person in the circle has to speak a word that rhymes with the one spoken by the leader. The aim is to make a complete chain of rhyming words that goes right round a circle (keep the groups small!).

Play *rhyming card games* using pictures of rhyming words. The pictures support those who may have difficulty in remembering or generating their own rhymes. Such cards can be used for pairs, snap, odd one out, happy families, dominoes and bingo, and can be incorporated into board games.

Many of the activities described in the section on rhythm and syllables (e.g. choral recitations) can be adapted to focus on rhyme.

Linking Rhyme to Reading and Writing

Rhyming stories and poems can be used as reading texts. Discuss the rhymes within them. Look at common letter patterns, and see how they usually rhyme. Encourage the learner to write down the rhyming words. The learner can mark rhyming words in printed poems with a highlighter pen. Delete some of the rhymes in a poem for the learner to write in either independently or through multiple choice.

Use *word cards and plastic letters* alongside the oral rhyming activities.

Encourage the *writing of poems and rhyming stories* in the writing corner. Create displays and anthologies—the learners love to have their writing used by others for reading texts. Within the corner designate an area of board as a rhyming area. Select a word a week—learners can pin rhyming words on the board, and they can be shared in a session at the end of the week. As a group, try writing a silly poem using the rhymes discovered.

Use a learner's *reading pack cards* (p.101) or the letters in the *alphabet rainbow* (p.90). Create rhyming words by changing initial sounds (onset and rime p.83). Write down the words created.

Use rhyme for working out unfamiliar words in *shared reading*. A word that has been refused (e.g. 'grain') can be illuminated by pointing out a similar, more familiar word (e.g. 'train'): "I expect you know this word. Can you use it to help?".

Follow up the oral games already described (e.g. make lists of written rhyming chains).

Developing Awareness of Alliteration

Recognizing when words begin with the same sound is an important step towards phonemic awareness. The technical term 'alliteration' does not have to be used. There are many games that can develop this awareness, many of them everyday, familiar ones.

Packs of picture cards are useful in creating a variety of games whose object is to sort and match words that begin with the same sound. Use the rules and formats of board games, snap, pairs, happy families, bingo, odd one out, dominoes, etc.

I Spy is an obvious choice, and can be adapted in many ways. Say: 'I spy with my little eye something beginning with the sound /s/ ...the same sound as cup ... the sound /s/, and it rhymes with bun ... the sound /m/, and it has two syllables'.

In this way you can also work on other aspects of phonological awareness.

In *The Minister's Cat*, learners have to think of adjectives beginning with the same sound. The leader starts the game by selecting a sound, e.g. /f/, and says 'The minister's cat is a fierce cat'. The next player could say "The minister's cat is a fat cat" and so on. If you feel that 'the minister' is too unfamiliar to your learners, try the caretaker's cat, or the policeman's cat.

Build up a store of *poems* that have alliterative words within them. Read them aloud, and draw attention to the alliteration.

Tongue twisters are popular, and usually rely on alliteration for their effect. Popular ones: 'Round and round the rugged rocks the ragged rascal ran'; 'Peter Piper picked a peck of pickled pepper'; 'She sells sea shells on the sea shore'. Learners enjoy developing their own.

Use a *'feely bag'*. Younger children enjoy identifying objects in the bag. The objects all begin with the same sound, and the sound can then be actively used as a clue.

Have an *interest table* in the classroom that has collections of objects that begin with the same sound.

Play *Kim's Game*: put a collection of objects on a tray, each beginning with the same sound. Cover the objects, and secretly remove one of them. The learner has to look again at the tray and identify the missing object.

Make a *story box*. Collect objects beginning with the same sound, and put them in a box. Take them out one by one and discuss them. The players can then make up a story that uses the objects as part of the narrative.

Sort objects by sound. The learner can be given a collection of things to sort according to their first sound. Pictures can be used instead of objects.

"I went shopping and I bought..." can be linked to a common initial sound. The players can buy in turn sausages, sweets, satsumas, etc. Be prepared for items such as 'celery' to appear; this is quite correct if the activity is based on sound alone. If spelling and writing are involved, it may be the moment to talk about exceptions to rules.

Collect magazine pictures of objects beginning with the same sound and stick them in a scrapbook or on a wall display. Make sure the learner has access to these by storing them in the writing or library corner.

Linking Alliteration to Reading and Writing

Use the environment. Look for words that begin with the same sound in labels, shop signs, notices, and when sharing books. Discuss them and point out that the same letter is often used. Soon learners will begin to notice them for themselves: "Look, that word begins with the same letter as my name!'

The learner can *highlight words* that begin with a chosen sound, using a photocopied page from a familiar book. The words could then be written down by the learner.

Make lists: many emergent writers love writing lists. Suggest lists of things that begin with the same sound, e.g. make a shopping list of things that begin with /t/. Picture word cards or simple dictionaries can give spelling support.

Adapt 'The Minister's Cat' to include writing. In the writing corner, put up a picture of the cat (or another animal) and suggest written descriptions of the animal using words beginning with the chosen sound. Share the texts with the whole class, and use them for reading.

Make a copy of a *group story* or news item. Choose a sound and highlight words within the story. Leave the piece displayed for rereading.

Tongue twisters and 'story box' activities are obvious choices for writing activities. Save and use the outcomes. The learning will be all the more successful as it is based on the learners' own thoughts, ideas, and shared experiences.

Wooden or plastic letters can be linked to most alliteration activities to emphasize the link between sound and letter shape. Let the learners trace over textured letters, and write them in the air, on paper and in sand. In this way learning becomes truly multisensory as the words are spoken and heard, the initial sound identified, and the corresponding letter shape seen and written.

Developing Awareness of Onset and Rime

Learners can easily identify initial sounds, but find it much more difficult to discriminate and sequence sounds in the middle and at the end of a word. Working on a word or syllable that has two parts—a beginning (initial consonant or consonant blend) and an ending (the vowel plus the final consonant or consonant blend) is not so demanding on the learner. Phoneme awareness training demands fine sound discrimination, and greater sequencing ability. Thus identification of onset and rime is a useful step between identification of syllables, and identification of individual sounds within the syllables. Training in awareness of onset and rime helps the learner to develop the strategy of use of analogy in reading.

Use oral blending: ask the learner: "Can you tell what word I am thinking of?" Then present a word with a one second gap between onset and rime. Say the sounds very purely, with no added /er/ sounds—/s/ is 'sss', not 'ser'. Begin with simple sounds, and move onto more complex ones. For example:

1.   c-at, b-ag, k-ick, h-en, d-ot, g-un, r-un, w-in.
2.   l-ost, s-and, j-ump, b-ang, w-ish, s-oft, d-esk.
3.   st-ar, gl-ass, fr-og, dr-um, gr-ape, cl-ock, sw-eet.
4.   sp-end, sh-ark, pr-ince, cr-isp, ch-est, br-ush.

Present this type of activity within the context of listening to a short paragraph from a story or rhyme. Ask the learner to complete the words as you wait: "Mary had a little l......, its fl........ was white as sn........." etc. Once the learner has got the idea use less familiar extracts.

Generate new words. Choose a particular rime (e.g. -at, -in, -ake) and see if the learner can make new words by adding different onsets. The words can be supplied by the learners, or the teacher can add various onsets and ask the learners to judge if they make a real or nonsense word.

Play group games. Divide a class group into two sets. Each person in the first set has to secretly choose an onset. Each person in the second set has to think of a rime. On a signal the players have two minutes to move round the room to find a partner to make a whole word. The only sounds that may be made as the partners look for a partner are the sound of the onset and rime they have selected.

Segment words. Breaking whole words into onset and rime chunks is a slightly harder task than blending. Ask the learner: "Can you say this word in two bits- the beginning, then the ending?" You will need to say the word very clearly, perhaps emphasising initial blends.

Linking Onset and Rime Activities to Reading and Writing

Work from the *alphabet rainbow* (see p.90) arranged in front of the learner. Make a rime (e.g. 'and') from the letters. The learner finds different onsets and puts them in front of the rime, blending them to make a word. Include some nonsense words to ensure that the learner is blending, and not just relying on sight vocabulary. The reading pack can be used in a similar way. Make a written list of the words produced, practising joined handwriting. Tick the ones that are real words. Discuss their meaning and include them in sentences that are to be read.

A pairs game can be made with cards of two colours. Print a selection of onsets onto one colour of card, and a selection of rimes on the other colour. Turn all the cards face down. Turn over one onset card and one rime card. Put them together and read them. If they make a real word, the player keeps the pair and has one more turn. If they make a nonsense syllable, the player puts them back and the next player has a turn.

Two piece jigsaws of words cut into onset and rime can be made. These can have the added support of a picture if needed.

Make a *fishing game* out of card, magnets on string, and paper clips. The players fish for onsets and rimes and score points for making whole words.

Use *board games*. Print one-syllable words onto the squares of a board game. Each time the learner lands on a word, it has to be segmented into onset and rime in order to gain a counter from the kitty. The first player to reach the end of the board has two free counters. The player with the most counters is the winner.

Use *shared reading*. Encourage the use of onset and rime division when attempting unfamiliar words in reading. Ask the learner to mark the vowel with a pencil, and to identify the rime that follows. Now see if the whole word can be read by blending together the onset and rime. Two or more syllable words can be worked out in the same way by splitting them into syllables first (see p.80). Make sure that the learner has the skills to succeed at the words you choose—'stand' should only be attempted when 'st' is in the reading pack, and 'and' has been introduced as a rime in other activities. The learner will have to be very far on in the structure before you can be confident that a word like 'search' is accessible to analysis. A word like 'laugh' never will be.

Use *spelling tests*. Give lists of words to be learned for reading or spelling. Include words with common onsets or rimes to reinforce the letter sound pattern. Display them in the classroom or the writing corner. Link this to handwriting practice. Test at the end of the week.

Encourage the use of onsets and rimes in *invented spelling* and 'best guess' days. Remind the learners when they ask for spellings that consist of onsets and rimes they have covered.

Write *poems, limericks and jingles*, looking for opportunities to reinforce skills teaching on onset and rime.

Make a *Word Slide* based on onset and rime:

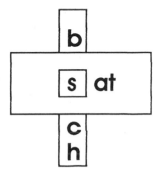

Figure 8.1 A Word Slide

Use *plastic or wooden letters* in the oral activities. Write down the words that are made.

Developing Phonemic Awareness

When the learner is able to detect rhyme and alliteration, to divide words into syllables, and to divide words into onset and rime, it is time to focus on single phonemes. The learner needs to identify single sounds made, not only at the beginning of words, but also in the middle and at the end. Growing skills enable the learner to blend a whole sequence of sounds into words, or to segment words into constituent sounds.

Concrete aids cut out a great deal of confusing verbal explanation, and reduce the load on short-term memory. An approach used in *Reading Recovery* (Clay, 1993b) and in *Sound Linkage* (Hatcher, 1994) is useful. The learner has a strip of card marked into a row of three squares. Each square denotes a phoneme. The learner is asked if a particular sound comes at the beginning, middle or end of a word, and to place a counter in the appropriate square. This exercise also checks that the learner understands the concept of beginning, middle and end. If not, specific work should be carried out in this area first. (Hatcher's 1994 programme has useful work in this area.) Word-finding difficulties can make it hard for the

learner to verbalize the correct labels, even if they do understand the concept—
"start...er.. middle.. I mean end" is a typical verbal response. The use of the card
removes the complication of recall and articulation of labels, as well as underlining the right to left sequence of our letter sound code. The same card technique
can be used to count the number of phonemes in words. The learner listens to a
word, then places one counter for each phoneme onto a square. The strips of card
should not indicate the answer by their length—make them a couple of squares
longer than necessary. Phonemes can also be counted by tapping or clapping.

Ask the learner to listen to two words spoken clearly by the teacher, and to say
if they begin with the *same sound* (e.g. cat, car; pin, bed). Use the same routine for
end and middle sounds.

Listen for the *'odd one out'*. Speak a sequence of three words and ask the learner
to listen to the end sounds and say which one is the odd one out (e.g. cat, jam, sum;
pet, bit, dog). This work can be supported by pictures to help learners with a poor
short-term memory.

Generate *word chains*. Ask the learner to say a word beginning or ending with
the same sound as a word you have spoken. Play this with a group in a circle,
trying to complete the chain without a break.

Practise *blending phonemes together* to make a word. Ask the learner: "Can you tell
what word I am thinking of?" Then present a word with a one second gap
between each phoneme, e.g. c-a-t, cr-a-sh. Start with two phonemes, and build up
very gradually. Blending can be very difficult for some learners, so don't go too
fast (see Hatcher, 1994, for ideas).

Try *phoneme deletion*. Ask the learner to miss off a sound from the beginning of a
word, and say what is left: "Take the /d/ off dog, what is left?" The answer ('-og')
is a nonsense syllable, and very difficult for some learners to handle. This is a
complex task, and is particularly difficult when the sound deleted comes at the
end of a word (e.g. 't' from 'hat' leaves 'ha') and interferes with the natural onset
and rime division.

Linking Phoneme Awareness to Reading and Writing

The oral activities described above can be reinforced through the use of letter
shapes, tracing the letters in the air and writing them down. Remember, for the
learning to be truly multisensory the learner must see the letter, feel the shape of it
being written, say the sound, feel the sound being articulated in the mouth and
hear it. These links cannot be stressed enough. We want the links to be automatic—not 'known' or 'recognized', but built into the body and available for
recall as reflex responses.

Use the *structure* beginning on p124 to teach the letter sounds. The reading pack
routines on p.101 are essential to this learning. There are strong links with the
alphabet work (p.88) as the learner comes to realise that the letters have both names
and sounds.

Using *current texts* (reading books, poems, newspapers, etc.), focus on a particular sound. Highlight a chosen letter with marker pens, and discuss its position within a word, and the sound it makes. This sort of activity often throws up something unexpected (e.g. 'c' at the beginning of 'circle'). Make a list of the marked words. Display the marked texts for future study.

Find opportunities in *shared reading* activities to look for sounds that are the focus of skills teaching. Carry out this activity after a passage has been read and enjoyed so that the meaning and flow of the piece remain intact. Remind the learner to use letter–sound knowledge when attacking unfamiliar words in independent reading.

Use the *learner's own writing*. The best links of all are made through writing and redrafting activities. Encourage invented spellings; in this activity, the learners truly make their skills work for them (see p.69).

Play games: play letter–sound pairs, snap, dominoes, bingo, happy families. Use a mix of pictures, letters and written words in these games. Play games that concentrate on the beginning, middle or end sound. Reinforce terms such as letter, sound, word, beginning, middle, end. Adapt board games to include letter–sound knowledge.

Cut up words: print whole words on paper for the learner to read, then to cut into phonemes. They enjoy preparing these as jigsaws for friends to complete and read.

Use nonsense words: athough we would always strongly advocate the importance of reading for meaning, we would suggest that you sometimes work with nonsense words as well as real words. Some learners are so distracted by the search for meaning that they do not utilise the letter–sound knowledge they have. By blending together such sequences as 'c-o-n' or 'sp-o-d', they are able to concentrate on rehearsing their blending and segmentation skills. Nonsense rhymes can be created from some of these words for others to read.

Chapter 9:
The Alphabet

Alphabet Knowledge

Before children are ready to use letter sound relationships, they can be taught to identify the letters as familiar objects (see Adams, 1990 for a review of research evidence on the importance of alphabet knowledge as a predictor of reading ability; also her account of the need for ease of recognition of individual letters). Knowledge of letters can affect all areas of reading and writing; words, sentences, stories, are made from familiar components, and familiarity can help the learner to notice their appearance in text. Observation increases knowledge, and use of skills can become an integral part of the pleasurable experience of sharing a book. Increasing ability to identify letters as objects is useful when the learner reaches the stage of adding in the extra layer of letter–sound link. Whatever methods are appropriate for the rote learning of any information can be used.

There are certain decisions that have to be made before one can focus on teaching methods:

Names or Sounds?

Readers use letter sounds when reading or writing. The only time that letter names are habitually used is when someone is asked to spell a word, for example, "How do you spell your name?". However, there are some strong motives for teaching letter names:

1. One letter can have many sounds (think of 'a' in apple, acorn, arch, banana); one sound can have many spellings (think of the /k/ sound in cat, king, chemist, antique). The name is consistent, though children who have watched American educational programmes such as Sesame Street may call the letter z 'zee'.
2. Children being taught skills need to be accorded the respect of being given the correct label. Using 'nicknames' like 'curly /k/ and kicking/k/' seems to the authors an unnecessary and patronizing approach—and adds yet another thing to disentangle.

3.   Learning the correct label gives the learner control and mastery over the object. As Adams (1990) points out, "there is, in itself, pedagogical power in having a label for a to-be-learned concept". Just learning that a letter has a name is in itself a useful piece of metalinguistic knowledge.

4.   Even children with language-poor backgrounds have usually come across some of the letter names. ABC books, posters, nursery songs will have used letter names. Unless the names are firmly fixed, they will be a source of confusion rather than elucidation. Just take one example—think of the nexus of confusion surrounding the names and sounds of the letters U, W and Y. The name of Y starts with the sound made by the letter W; the name of the letter U starts with the sound made by the letter Y; the name of the letter U is found in the name of W. No wonder they so frequently provide a major stumbling-block to beginner readers and writers. When children start to invent their own spellings (Read, 1986), they often use a letter to signify a syllable (see Nicholas's letter in Chapter 2, p.18)—this is a great step forward in freedom of communication through writing, but a strong signal that letter/name confusion has to be tackled at some time.

5.   Using the correct labels for the letters will heighten the learner's sensitivity to minute and critical differences in the formation of the letters, and encourage an ability to notice and make fine discriminations. Lower-case 'b' and 'd' are only differentiated through their spatial orientation, a pretty meaningless distinction to a child who has not yet settled to choosing a dominant eye or hand. Progress is begun when the letter name 'd' begins to collect together all its various forms and fonts, including the upper-case forms that are more distinctively different.

Our experience is that learning letter names can be a pleasant and rewarding activity, and the learning can precede or run concurrently with teaching on sound–symbol correspondence. Most of the letter names contain an indication of that letter's sound; this can be a mixed blessing, as the letter names can be a source of confusion to children with language difficulties, including severe word-finding difficulties, or extensive articulation problems. Such children may benefit from an approach like cued articulation (see p.37), which can be worked out with a communication therapist. However, it is very comforting to realise that, on one level, all the complexities of the English language can be reduced to 26 individual units!

Lower or Upper Case?

Upper case letters have the advantage of being distinctive and, on the whole, consistent. Much of the adult world is marked in capitals—DANGER, EXIT, STOP, TESCO. Lower case letters have the disadvantages of being dependent on specific orientation (d,b,p,q), and of varying in relation to the base line. But most of the print that children will read is lower case, and the lower case letter form the basis for joined handwriting, which the child will eventually use as its method of written communication. It is important that children (and their teachers!) do not fall into the trap of thinking that the upper case represents the name, and the lower case the sound. The authors' opinion is that initial teaching is best approached using lower case, and adding in upper case later. Older children, receiving a remedial programme, are usually taught using upper case. But the authors are not aware of any research that confirms these opinions.

Teaching the Letter Names

Use wooden or plastic letters—Galt make some lovely big wooden ones, and many toy shops and educational suppliers provide letters that are pleasant to handle.

Lay out the letters in an arc on a table in alphabetical order, as if resting on a rainbow, so that all the letters are equidistant from the learner's hand. For younger children, considerable support in producing the alphabet sequence is required. This can be achieved through:

1.   Matching a second set of letters onto a set arranged by the teacher.
2.   Matching onto an alphabet rainbow made from drawing round the letter shapes.
3.   Sharing the load with a teacher, taking it in turn to place the letter shapes.
4.   Using a wall frieze or an alphabet book as a guide to work from.

Other activities include:

1.   Printing alphabets with paint and letter shapes or rubber stamps and ink.
2.   Drawing round letter shapes to produce an alphabet.
3.   Tracing over, colouring or decorating pre-prepared alphabets, naming the letters in sequence.
4.   Cutting out letters and sticking them in sequence, using letters prepared by the teacher or cut from newspapers or magazines.
5.   Fishing for magnetic letters using a magnet on the end of a string and placing your catch in sequence.
6.   Using computer programs such as *My World* (SEMERC) that include alphabet sequencing.

When lower case letters can be sequenced, try matching capitals to lower case or vice versa.

Young pupils can enjoy play with letters and the alphabet sequences through inset trays, alphabet jigsaws, interlocking letters, feely letters, alphabet building blocks, etc. Such play, through the tactile experiences of feeling, arranging and drawing round letters, adds a further dimension to visual familiarity with their shapes through naming and looking. Some of these materials can be used with older pupils but always take care that age-appropriate activities and materials are used.

A full alphabet does not always have to be produced; indeed 26 letters can be overwhelming for some pupils. A small selection of letters with very different shapes may be an ideal starting point, or use part of the alphabet, for example A to E.

Alphabet Activities for the Older Learner

The older learner can have a brisker introduction to the alphabet arc. Initially the teacher's help might be required, but the learner will gradually take over more and more of the task as confidence and knowledge increase. Explain that M and N are at the top of the arc; learners often know A,B,C, and X,Y,Z. Explain that the letter names never change; only Z has an American pronunciation (zee). Some letters will have been given nicknames, like curly /k/ and kicking /k/, but we are going to use the real names.

When the letters are becoming familiar, vary the task; put the letters in a bag, ask the learner to extract them with eyes shut, and identify by feel. Then open the eyes, and place the letters in approximately the right place on the table, gradually building up the arc without relying on alphabetical order.

Some learners like to use a stop watch to time themselves in setting out the alphabet.

Learning the Letter Names

1.   The learner touches each letter in turn. Teacher and learner say the alphabet together.
2.   Say the whole alphabet in pairs, with the accent on the second: AB/, CD/, EF/. Put the accent on the first of the pair: A/B, C/D, etc. Say in threes, varying the accent: A,B,C/ D,E,F/, etc.
3.   Say the alphabet with the same rhythm and accent as a learner's name, e.g. Da/vid, A/B, C/D. Catherine is A/BC, D/EF etc. Use car names: Mercedes is AB/C, DE/F etc.
4.   Sing the alphabet. It can be fitted into various tunes (e.g. Twinkle twinkle little star)

Use the Arc to Teach Alphabetical Order

Many learners find it difficult to master any sequence. Rather than spending time repeating verbal lists, use the sequence for activities that will reinforce and add to their knowledge.

1.   Learner closes eyes; teacher names a letter; learner points to the right area of the alphabet. Or you can remove a letter, and adjust the spaces. Then the learner has to open the eyes and decide which letter is missing.
2.   Play the shopping game with a group in a circle. The first player says, "I went to the shop and I bought an apple"; the next one could buy a book, a

cat..., etc. To vary the game, and to increase opportunities for social inter-
action, suggest that the circle members quote the purchase of the preceding
player: "John bought an apple. I bought a book." "Emma bought a book. I
bought a cat".

3.   Use the letters for strengthening auditory and visual short-term memory.
        Try naming two letters and ask the learner to repeat the names, take the
        letters out of the arc, and line them up in the same order. To start with, you
        will have to choose letters that you know the learner is sure of; you may also
        need to help the learner visually locate the letters within the arc. You may
        need to present the letters on cards, so that there is a visual check; as confi-
        dence increases, the learner will be able to look at the card and name the
        letters without the teacher's help. Move on to three, then four, then five.
        When you reach six, it is a good idea to teach strategies like dividing the six
        into two groups of three.

All the activities and games described are more fun if the roles of teacher and
learner are passed around—sometimes the adult can be 'tested' by the child, or
learners can 'test' each other. Children who have been struggling for years to
commit the alphabet to memory amaze themselves and their parents by their
success when following such a regular programme. Instead of concentrating on
trying to learn the sequence, they are using it, and having fun. It is so much easier
to learn something when you are relaxed. Many of these activities were first experienced in the early 1970s by one of the authors as a young teacher on Kathleen
Hickey's course at the Dyslexia Institute in Staines, and her learners are still
enjoying them!

Using Dictionaries

A dictionary is a wonderful tool for learning about language, and for developing
use of language. It is not merely an answer book that tells you how to use, spell, or
pronounce a word. Different dictionaries have different purposes, and each new
volume has to be explored. In exploring them, skills and strategies need to be
developed.

Lexicographers select their diacritical markings from a common pool, but they
choose the ones that are appropriate to the purpose of the dictionary. Thus each
particular dictionary needs careful inspection—do read the introductions. All
dictionaries use the same alphabetical order, and the activities described on the
preceding pages (p.90-92) will increase familiarity with this order.

Choosing a Dictionary

Home-made dictionaries. As children ask for words to be spelled for writing, they can
be entered into a small exercise book, using a different page for each letter. A
useful routine is to try out the word on a piece of scrap paper, thus giving the child
an opportunity to practise inventing spellings (see p.69), then to decide with the
child whether the word is important enough to be entered into the spelling dictio-

nary— it is an important word if it is likely to be used again. Children who are just beginning to link sound with letter can have a clue word to illustrate each section—the clue words can be the familiar ones used in the reading pack.

Spelling dictionaries. A simple spelling dictionary without definitions can be useful in developing early skills in looking up words, and give the child an opportunity to check a guess. *Spell It Yourself* (Hawker, 1962) is easy to use. An index gives the page of words with the same first two letters. Only the base words are listed in bold type, with the suffixes in lighter type, and an indication of the way the suffix is added (final letter doubled, silent 'e' dropped, or 'y' changed to 'i'). No definitions are included, but homophones are indicated. Its clear presentation eases the task of the poor reader in scanning the page for a particular word. The user has to exercise sound processing skills, dividing the word into syllables, isolating and ordering the sounds within the syllables. The learner is given experience in using alphabetical order within the word, rather than having to listen to confusing explanations of how it works. Its small vocabulary, and its cursory indication of homophones, limits its usefulness for independent use. *The ACE Spelling Dictionary* (Mosely and Nicol, 1986) uses an index that is purely sound based—an Aurally Coded English dictionary. To find a word, the user identifies the vowel sound of the first syllable, finds the index, finds a picture that matches the vowel sound, identifies the first letter of the word, and is then referred to the correct page. On that page, the words are sorted into categories according to the number of syllables, and the user has only to scan down a single column. It is complicated to introduce, and demands a good level of sound processing and organizational skills, but can be used independently and has an extensive vocabulary.

Most publishers have small volumes that list only the words for spelling, often distinguishing homophones by colour or by font.

General purpose dictionaries. Choose a dictionary that is clearly set out, and aimed at an appropriate age group. The Oxford Primary School Dictionary (Augarde 1993) is an example of a book that is easy to use, and will help to develop strategies that are needed to explore a wide range of dictionaries. The first and last headword on each double page is printed boldly at the top of each page. Each headword is defined, giving examples of usage where necessary, and simple syntactical information is given. Language register is indicated where a usage is informal or slang. Pronunciation is conveyed by simple phonics (e.g. Christmas: say krist-mas) or by rhyming words (draughts rhymes with crafts). The breve is used to indicate a short vowel sound.

All this information needs to be studied with the child, so that the poor reader is not confused, and that study needs to be repeated with each different dictionary.

Finding a word. Augur and Briggs (1992) describe Hickey's a thoughtful approach that recognizes the stages that a learner has to go through in tracking down one word hidden amongst thousands.

Look at the particular volume being used, and work out how the words are distributed. Open the volume at three points: the quarter, half, and three-quarter points. Notice which words fall into which section. Instead of making the alphabet arc, you can arrange the wooden or plastic letters to correspond with the distribution of the dictionary you are using. For example, The Oxford opens as follows:

A B C D
E F G H I J K L
M N O P Q R
S T U V W X Y Z

Hickey refers to these uneven quarters as quartiles. You can invent a mnemonic to remind you of the starting letters of the quartiles of your particular dictionary (e.g. All Elephants Munch Sausages; Avoid Examining Melancholy Skunks).

Once the child is familiar with the distribution of the words, challenge each other to open the volume at a page where the words begin with a certain letter. Start with easy ones like 's', and notice how some letters are more popular than others in starting words. As skills develop, you can aim to find a specific word with a limited number of openings of the book. Hickey suggests aiming for five openings. Such a limitation has an effect of encouraging the child to plan each move carefully, thus identifying and internalizing the process of finding a word, and eliminating the habit of optimistic but fruitless flipping through the pages.

Chapter 10:
A Structured Approach

Introduction to Sound–Symbol Links

When to Begin

Learners can enjoy books as soon as they can understand language, and they can begin to play with letters and learn their names as soon as they understand the purpose of print. Embarking on systematic instruction in linking sounds with letters or letter clusters has to be considered carefully. Successful learners tune into reading through a holistic learning process that is as complex as the human mind, and part of the individual's development of language. They first become interested in sound symbol links when they need to invent spellings (see p.69), and this is as good a time as any to embark on a systematic, structured introduction to the letters so that the links between sound, shape, and hand movement are clear and free from confusion. As the links begin to be formed for writing, some children spontaneously carry the knowledge over to reading, and begin to vocalize the initial sounds of an unfamiliar word. Others will need to be led to using the strategy, 'Look, I think you know how that word begins—do you remember the sound that letter makes? Say the sound, and see if it gives you a clue'.

Where to Begin

The multisensory structured methods described here are diagnostic. Each link between looking, saying, writing, hearing, and sequencing needs to be tested. Going through the routines tests each link; if the learner already 'knows' the sound, good; we won't need to spend much time on it. However, 'knowing' is not the same as being able to use in reading and writing. The knowledge is not usable until the learner can have an automatic, speedy response to the stimulus of a letter or a letter cluster. A thorough, structured introduction to each little piece of knowledge builds in these responses, and enables the learner to integrate these fragments into a mental database. New strategies give the learner the ability to gather up bits of information that were half understood, and they also become organized into usable networks; the piles of bricks that have been lying about on the building site start to become walls. So start at the beginning. The pace and emphasis will vary according to need.

The necessary overlearning is taken care of by simple, repetitive, self-checking routines. The letter(s) are introduced one by one, and collected into a pack that is practised regularly. The routines exercise the links between sound and symbol. A stimulus is presented to ears or to eyes, and the learner responds by making a sound that they hear and feel, and/or a hand movement that they feel, to make a letter that they see.

The purpose of daily repetition of the routines is not to test the learner's knowledge; it is to strengthen the links between sound and symbol. The links are truly internalized when they are used spontaneously in holistic literacy activities.

Introducing a New Phonogram

A phonogram is a letter or group of letters representing a sound.

Each link between sound and symbol needs to be checked (we shall use the letter 'p' as an example). Ask, rather than tell the learner—'Do you know the name of this letter?' 'Yes, its name is p'.

Use the multisensory teaching routine: *see-hear-say-write*.

Can the learner *see* the letter, and recognize it in its various forms? Identify upper and lower case examples, using a variety of books, posters, newspapers, and cursive handwriting. Computers and word processors provide examples of various fonts—print selections of letters, and ask the learner to ring every 'p'.

Can the learner *hear* the sound that letter makes? Ask the learner to listen to some words, and identify the ones that start with the /p/ sound. (e.g. pin/pig/dog; plan/clap/play; pest/best—notice the increasing difficulty of the task). Can the learner identify the position of the /p/ sound; beginning, middle or end of the word? (pot, price, happy, step, paper).

Can the learner *say* the sound? Seek the help of a communication therapist when working out an approach for learners with major articulation problems. Learners with minor problems (e.g. f/th, w/r, s/th confusion) will need help in pronouncing the sound more accurately. These learners must be made aware of their difficulties, and helped to develop strategies that maximize use of visual memory in these problem areas. Cued articulation is a wonderful tool for helping the learner to focus on, and repeat, the sound correctly.

Can the learner *write* the letter? An automatic, fluent hand movement for each letter, and each joining, relieves the memory load. For some learners, the hand movement is a source of strength, providing the learner with a cue.

Handwriting

Many approaches to spelling emphasize the importance of writing, instructing the learners to Look, Cover, Write, Check when learning a spelling pattern or a new word. A structured multisensory programme gives the learners an opportunity to build into their bodies an automatic, fluent hand movement for each letter and each spelling pattern. It is important to link hand movement to sound. If learners

have a pleasant, clear and fluent handwriting, the routines are still important—
the handwriting is for them a strength that can be used as a memory trigger.

Style: Print or Joined Writing?

The learner will always have print presented as the main medium for reading,
though the font will vary enormously depending on the material presented (shop
fronts, posters, newspapers, early readers etc.). As soon as the learner is ready to
adopt phonic strategies for word synthesis, it seems logical to link the sound with
the hand movement that will become their mature form of expression. They will
still need to use print of various kinds for graphic effect in writing for different
purposes.

The style used (figure 10.1) here is a simple, unornamented cursive style. Its
base is the printed form, which most infant teachers would accept as 'normal'.
Each letter or letter cluster follows the same guidelines:

1.   Start from the baseline with an approach stroke.
2.   Move to the starting point of the printed letter.
3.   Complete the letter.
4.   Form a leaving stroke that can connect with the approach stroke of the next
     letter.

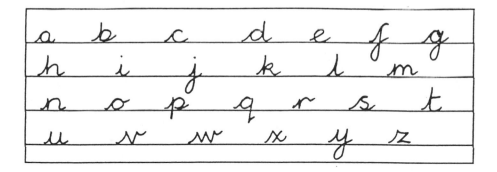

Figure 10.1 Handwriting style

This particular style is not obligatory—the letter form can be varied according
to taste, as long as the pen does not have to be lifted in the middle of a word. This
means that some descenders (f, g, j and y) will have loops, an unpleasant reminder
for some older teachers of strict training methods of the past. But adoption of
these simple generalities can solve many problems caused by short-term memory
weakness and sequencing confusion, resulting in reversals and inversions of letters
and words:

1.   The memory load is lessened; all letters start from the base line. Joinings from
     letters that leave from the top (b, o, r, v and w) will need special attention.

2.   The direction of the letter is controlled by a movement stored in the body rather than in the conscious memory.
3.   The relationship between the letter and the base line is strengthened, so that the sections of the letters stay in the correct zones.
4.   Spaces between words become distinct.

A few loops are a small price to pay for these advantages!

Although our approach to spelling is based on the learner developing a joined hand, this may not always be appropriate. For the youngest learners, making the link between letters and a word written in a joined hand, and print typefaces in books, can add extra complications and confusion to the learning process. Some learners may not see any connections between the styles. It may be more appropriate to teach an initial print consisting of the basic shapes within the joined form. This can then be developed into a joined style when the learner is ready.

Older learners and their teachers may also decide that the effort of mastering a new handwriting style is not worth the trouble. Sometimes the learner has an attractive and speedy print, and does not want to add in joinings. Sometimes there are time constraints—exams coming up, or a move to secondary school. Just make a decision about letter formation, and link the hand movement with the sound it makes, how it feels in the mouth, and its appearance.

Capitals (figure 10.2) are usually printed though a few letters (e.g. C, K, E) can reach the approach stroke of the next letter.

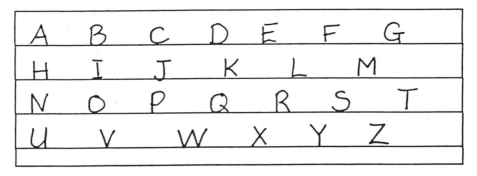

Figure 10.2 Capital letters.

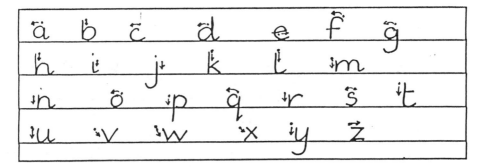

Figure 10.3 Basic print (lower case)

The basic print recommended is set out in figure 10.3. We have a preference for teaching letters with leaving strokes if appropriate to the learner. The transfer to a joined hand is then made more smoothly.

Multisensory Handwriting Routines

If a learner is to build a letter–sound link into the body, it is not enough to involve only ears and eyes. Movement is also important. The learner needs to be aware of the air moving from the lungs, and being shaped by tongue, lips and throat. Another area of mastery is in learning the correct hand movement for each link. As the learner moves through the structure, mastering the hand movement becomes easier. Hickey describes a simple routine that is adequate for most learners. (To start with, the phonograms are individual letters. As the learner moves through the structure, some sounds require two or more letters—th, sh, igh etc. The routines are the same.)

Look: the teacher prints a large letter on a blackboard, and shows how the written form relates to the printed form. Start from the base line—approach to the start of the printed letter; write the letter; form a leaving stroke.

Trace: learners trace over the teacher's letter repeatedly until they are confident. While writing, say the sound and then the name of the letter.

Copy: learners copy the letter, repeating sound and name, then decide for themselves if there are any ways they could improve it.

Write from memory: if there are any problems at this stage, go back to tracing and copying.

Write with eyes shut: at this stage, any residual problems will reveal themselves.

This routine strengthens the link between the sound of the letter, its feel in the mouth, its movement, and its appearance. It completes the multisensory links between visual, auditory and kinesthetic modalities.

Kinesthetic Training

Some learners, particularly those with weakness in motor control, need more detailed practice before they can master the body movement and link it with the other aspects of the letter. It is sometimes necessary to take the learner's arm and guide it repeatedly through the correct movement, making sure of mastery in that area before bringing other modalities into play. Some learners need a great deal of practice. Using a variety of materials and approaches stops the necessary overlearning becoming tedious.

Trace in salt or sand.
Trace over velour letters.
Write on each other's backs.
Write in the air.
Use flipchart markers on large sheets of paper or newsprint.
Use whiteboards.
Trace on Hessian, silk etc.

Using Joined Handwriting

The next stage is to relate the routines above to pencil or pen and paper. For most learners, simple routines suffice. Books with 'tramlines' are a useful tool—Philip and Tacey have an exercise book with 4 mm and 12 mm ruling (Cambridge, ruling 9) that seems to suit most learners.

Write the letter in the books, and suggest that the learner traces, copies three times, and ticks the best. Then the learner and teacher can discuss the learner's choice, and see if they agree. If there are major problems at this stage, praise the effort, move onto something else, and come back to that letter on another occasion. The Spelling Pack routines will ensure that this letter will be practised regularly, and the multisensory links tested and strengthened. The word spelling routines will ensure that all the joinings are introduced and practised regularly.

Once a learner has started the process of modifying a handwriting style, there is inevitably a gap before the whole alphabet is covered. The handwriting sessions are focused on establishing the sound–symbol links, and the learner is practising sequencing of sounds in words for reading and writing, using word lists and short sentences that contain only the sounds covered. Meanwhile, in general reading and writing tasks, the learner will still be using well established techniques, including print. Sometimes learners will begin to include some of the joinings into their free writing. This can make their written work a bit more messy for a while, but should be discussed with others involved in the learner's education, and seen as a necessary development. Most of them treat their developing writing almost as an art form, as if they were learning italic lettering for graphic design.

The transfer of new handwriting skills into everyday writing has to be engineered deliberately and formally.

1. Discuss with the learner, and with other interested parties. Explain that, now that the alphabet is finished, every English word can be written, and that is going to be the normal form of expression. Print of various sorts will only be needed for graphic effect; for free writing, the cursive letter forms that have been linked with the sounds will be used.

2. In the exercise book normally used by the learner, draw 'tramlines' above the existing lines. Choose a height that suits the learner's normal style.

3. Make sure that the first few tasks are not too demanding—copying a poem, or copying a cloze text, will help the learner to concentrate on the handwriting style.

4. The first free writing tasks should be simple and make limited demands. When speed, automaticity and fluency are building up, then you can afford to start including demands on the learner's creativity, and expect stories or accounts of experience to be written in cursive writing.

5. Don't let the learner forget how to print—make sure that the skill is exercised through the production of posters, book titles, etc.

Building a Reading Pack: Essential Routines

The routines described here have been developed from the Hickey reading and spelling pack (Augur and Briggs 1992). The sound–letter links are accumulated gradually, and self-checking routines provide regular, relaxed practice, which exercises and strengthens the links between each stimulus and response. Some simple diacritical markings are used. The learner can be taught to use these markings, but their main purpose is to make things clear to a helper. All the learner really needs is the lower case and upper case example on the front of the card, and the picture on the back. The word and sound symbols are just a check, and provide a memo, telling the learners and helpers the exact response. In common with most dictionaries, the sound symbol is bracketed with oblique strokes.

1.	Short vowels: /ă/ as in cat (breve).
2.	Long vowels: /ā/ as in cake (macron).

Make sure that the learner can identify the letter by name, in its various written and printed forms, and can hear and say the sound.

Making a Reading Card

We use 2 × 3 inch cards, offcuts provided by a local printer. Learners who find such cards difficult to handle may need to use larger cards. We use pastel blue cards for vowels, and white cards for consonants. A third colour is useful for games and separate packs of rebus words, rimes, etc. The front and the back of each card is printed for you as each sound is introduced in the step-by-step programme.

Print the letter on the front of a card, lower and upper case. Print very neatly, offering the form that the learner is most likely to meet in reading books.

On the back of the card, print a clue word containing a clear example of the letter–sound link. A representation of the sound is printed after the word.

Draw a picture (learners usually prefer to draw their own) to provide an instant check. A glance at the picture is enough to trigger the word and sound; the learner does not have to be able to read the word, or decipher the bracketed sound.

When the handwritten form has been introduced, add it to the back of the card.

The learner looks at the front of the card, says the clue word and the sound, then turns the card over to check by looking at the picture. The front of the card is the stimulus, and the back provides the correct response. As the cards are accumulated, they are shuffled and practised in turn. If any mistake is made, the learner repeats the correct response, and puts the card to the back of the pack so that they can give it another turn. The pictures make the cards self-checking, though learners do enjoy saying the cards to each other. Even learners with word-finding difficulties find it possible to build up a number of responses quite quickly.

Daily Self-checking Reading Pack Routine

1. *Look* at front of card.
2. Remember and *say* clue word and sound.
3. Turn over to *check.*

An Alternative Reading Pack Routine

1. *Look* at the front of the card.
2. *Say* the sound (making the cued articulation sign if this support is being used).
3. Turn over to *check.*

Using the Cards as a Spelling Pack

Looking at the back of the card, the teacher says the sound in oblique brackets. The learner listens to the sound that the teacher has made, then repeats it, thus providing a model that is felt in the learner's mouth—it may not be pronounced in exactly the same way. Then the learner recalls the letter or letters that represent that sound. The sound is then spelled (i.e. the letter(s) are named), and written. If the learner has an alternative way of spelling that sound (e.g. 'c' and 'k' both represent the /k/ sound), the teacher should remember to mention the clue word: "/k/ as in cat?"

Sound Spelling Routine

1. *Listen* to the sound.
2. *Repeat* the sound.
3. *Name* the letter(s).
4. *Write* the letter(s). Add the hand-written form to the back of the reading card.

Word Reading and Word Spelling: Building Up a Sight Vocabulary

'Sight word reading' refers, not to a method of teaching by using flashcards, nor to the reading of irregular, difficult-to-spell words. Sight words are those words that can be instantly recognized (see Ehri, 1995). Skilled readers have formed connections for an enormous numbers of words, linking the written form with pronunciation and meaning.

Beginner readers will need to build up a starter vocabulary of sight words before the teacher embarks on a programme of phonic work. Young children need to understand the communicative nature of the printed word, have an understanding of the concept of words and letters, and be able to identify words logographically (see Frith, 1985 p.17) before analysing them in a more detailed way. Teachers should respond to this developmental process and help the young learner build up an initial sight vocabulary.

Some young learners will build up a sight vocabulary through sharing books and looking at environmental print in an informal way. Others will need a more structured and planned introduction.

The best words to target for this are those that will be the most motivating (and therefore the easiest) for the learner. Start with words relating to the learner's friends, family, home and school interests. Names of people are usually remembered first, along with names of easily imagined objects, or familiar verbs.

The words chosen can be incorporated into personal reading books made for individual learners, illustrated by the learners, or by photographs taken at school or supplied from home. The text should make use of the learner's own language, but should also be guided by the teacher so that the target vocabulary can be repeated. The learner is not expected to learn all the words in the text, just the targetwords. Draw attention to these words as the book is shared, commenting on links between words and letters in the text and those in the classroom (e.g. 'Look, that's the same as the word on the notice board; that word starts with the same letter as your name'). Some learners benefit from seeing the shape of the words drawn in outline.

Activities can be built around targetwords and personal reading books.

1. Sentence-matching strips can be made to match to the text. Cut them into words or sections and reassemble.
2. Word cards can be matched to the text.
3. When the text is familiar, cover it with a piece of paper, leaving the illustrations on view.
4. Ask the learner to arrange word cards into the appropriate sentences for the illustrations, then check.
5. Make a copy of the text, blanking out words to be filled in by the learner through cut and paste or by writing—you are in essence making an individualized cloze text.
6. Make games such as pairs, snap, dominoes, lotto, and snakes and ladders. They can use the targetwords and pictures representing them.
7. Trace over targetwords with fingers, coloured pens, in sand, etc.
8. Make the targetwords with plastic or wooden letters, and associate with the pictures that represent them.
9. Vary the context in which the words are experienced. Find them in other shared books, in classroom displays, etc. Initially the words may be recognized only in familiar contexts, but the learner will gradually come to understand that the word *cat* represents all cats, whatever the context.

We recommend that targetwords are learned *after* they have been presented in the meaningful context of a text, not before. It is also important to keep returning to the whole text. Words are much more easily learned within this supportive context. There is no expectation that the words should be learned before a personal book is used. Once the first book has become very familiar, make a second book that builds on and extends the vocabulary of the first. Incorporate these words into 'Breakthrough' folders (see p.72) and encourage the learners to use these words in their own writing.

Older learners can also enjoy personal readers. Choose a subject that interests them (cooking, pop music, soap operas, water sports, etc.), and use their enthusiasm for the subject. Be sensitive to the self-esteem of the older learner, perhaps presenting the exercise as a scrapbook related to the hobby or interest. They can help to prepare the captions to accompany drawings or cuttings. Use the computer to supply additional interesting graphics and fonts.

These ideas can easily be adapted to group work—the children in a class have much in common, and share many experiences and interest.

A skilled reader processes the words on the page so quickly that it seems they recognize all the words on the page at a glance. This is our aim for the learner with literacy difficulties. Our programme teaches phonic decoding skills, and encourages use of language cues. At the same time, we need to pay attention to a group of words that make up a large proportion of our language. Most of them are function words—words that bind the sentences together, whatever the topic of the piece of writing. Quick and automatic recognition and recall of these words can make reading much more fluent and pleasurable. It can also increase accuracy, which enables reading experience to become a foundation for increased success. Parents so often say about dyslexic children, "It's not the big words, it's the little words that cause the trouble". But the little function words are difficult to store for meaning, and their patterns are not so distinctive. It can be very difficult for a dyslexic learner to build in an accurate, reflex response, but it is well worth working at. Cobuild have given us permission to quote from The Bank of English, a computer store of over two hundred million words, that shows us which are the most frequent words found in spoken and written language. The first ten words make up more than a fifth of English—master those, and a fifth of everything you read will be transparent. Within our teaching programme we refer to these as keywords.

Learning a Keyword

In the structured list of sounds (p.124) we have included the 100 most common words (see table 10.1) as the letters are taught for writing. At this stage, the learner will be comfortably familiar with the letters, and have had experience of reading common onsets and rime patterns. The hundred keywords are included at this stage as irregular words to be learned. Learners can use tracing and writing as additional support for weak short-term memory when learning these words. Check that the learner can read and write the words in context and as isolated words.

Hundred most commonly used words

Table 10.1 Hundred most commonly used words (Cobuild) The Bank of English, November 1995)				
(1) 20.45%	(2) 5.95%	(3) 4.26%	(4) 2.90%	(5) 2.37%
the	was	by	's **	which
of	on	but	had	all
to	he	have	we	been
and	with	are	an	were
a	's *	they	there	she
in	you	from	or	who
that	as	his	one	so
it	I	this	said	would
is	be	not	will	up
for	at	has	their	her
(6) 1.96%	(7) 1.50%	(8) 1.33%	(9) 1.17%	(10) 0.98%
if	do	Mr.	him	very
about	new	my	well	years
what	people	after	your	most
more	like	just	know	think
when	now	year	then	get
out	some	first	I'm	may
can	time	over	last	back
no	them	only	also	says
two	than	other	me	any
its	into	could	because	our
's* (possessive); 's** (contraction)				

The 'look, say, cover, write, check' approach is common to many spelling schemes. Our approach to learning keywords is similar, but has to be more elaborate. It can be used with any keyword the learner has to learn. The learner with literacy difficulties has to be led through the 'look' stage very carefully. Learners with inconsistent, weak knowledge of any of the links between sound, shape and name of any of the 26 letters often have problems with essential sight words. Misreading *where* for *there*, or *what* for *want*, can destroy the meaning of a sentence and build in the learner insecurity and confusion. Adams reminds us of the way text is read letter by letter; it is important to look carefully at an individual letter in various fonts, and learn about it as a familiar object.

Look at the word. Is it easy to sound out? (e.g. is, and). Is there anything odd about it? (e.g. the 'f' in 'of' sounds like /v/; 'could' has silent letters). Is it like any other word already known? (e.g. 'there' and 'here' have opposite meanings, but share the same four letters).

Spell: repeat the letter names in order, first whilst looking at the word, then from memory.

Trace: write the word for the learner on the blackboard to be traced with finger or with chalk, or in large letters to be traced with highlighter or marker pen. The learner says the letter names as each letter is written.

Copy: write it for the learner in a book, and let the learner copy it, still spelling.

Write from memory: this can be done immediately after the copying stage, then a few minutes later, then added into the learner's 'test'. Add it to the learner's list of newly learned words, and 'test' it for reading and writing five or six times.

Reinforce new words through games and activities.

Transfer into reading and writing. Inform the class teacher when the learner is responsible for remembering a certain word. Set up a system of credits when the word is used and spelled correctly in free writing. Scan a newspaper or a reading book, highlighting the word.

Don't neglect the learner's own imagination and initiative. Ask if the learner can think of a good way to remember the word—sometimes their links can be surprising and effective.

Use of Rebus

The techniques described above can be supported by use of rebus symbols (see p.38, 75).

Games can be used to make the link between the symbol and the word, and to give extra practice in reading the words in isolation. Try:

Snap/pairs cards that contain a small selection of sight words. Include the written word alone, the symbol alone, and a combination of the two.

Lotto/dominoes, where symbols are matched to written words.

Board games such as snakes and ladders, which incorporate the reading of symbols and words.

Simple self-checking packs can be made for homework for individual practice in reading or spelling. Put the symbol on one side of the card, and the word on the other. The learner looks at the symbol, says or writes the word, then turns it over to check.

When the rebus symbol is a help rather than a hindrance (amazingly quickly in many cases!) pencil the symbol every time the word appears in a text. When the word is mastered, rub the symbol out.

Phonically Regular Words

At each step of the structure, as each new sound–symbol link is introduced or checked, the learner needs to practise sound blending in phonically regular words. When the learner is reading connected prose, we want the reader to have a range of strategies instantly available. Although instant recognition of the first letter–sound is a powerful and well used clue, sounding out a whole word only is one strategy amongst many. Sometimes it is useless—imagine trying to sound out a word like 'laugh'. But it can be a crucial technique, and one that dyslexic learners are likely to find particularly difficult. Regular practice in games and activities with single words give the learner growing facility without pushing this strategy into a dominant position in reading books.

In the step-by-step materials accompanying each stage of the structure, lists are provided that can be used to make games or practice packs. The simplest words, those that demand a simple level of phonological skill, have single consonants and one short vowel (e.g. sat, peg, tin, lot, bun). The next level includes initial consonant blends (e.g. crab, step, spin, stop, drug), or final consonant blends (e.g. hand, nest, lift, pond, dust). Consonant blends at the beginning and the end are a bit harder (e.g. stand, spend, crisp, blond, stump). Two and three syllable words are included for those learners who can handle syllable division as well as sound blending within the syllable. You might find that your learner will need to go all the way through the first stage of the structure at the simplest phonological level, then go back to add in practice at working out words at the next level of difficulty.

Using Onset and Rime Skills

If the learner can already orally divide words and syllables at the onset–rime boundary, the teacher will need to capitalize on that skill. If not, training in sound awareness, and practice in spotting 'chunks' of letters that rhyme, will encourage the learner to develop the strategy of use of analogy in reading. In spelling, handling two sound chunks rather than four or five helps a learner with poor short-term memory. It also helps them to remember the vowel; because the rime begins with a vowel, it becomes more prominent.

Onsets are presented on cards in the reading pack, and are practised regularly in the reading and spelling pack routines. As each new phonogram is introduced, the teacher will have to decide which of the possible rimes are appropriate and useful to the learner. Sometimes the rime will be judged to be important because there are a large number of high frequency words with a particular ending. Sometimes the rime will be part of a word that is important in a particular book, so that a child who keeps forgetting the word 'like' might work on words with an 'ike' ending. The only constraint is that all the letters of the rime should have been presented (p.96), so that the details of the individual letters are familiar in different contexts and fonts.

Using our letter order (see p.121) , the first five letters give four possible rimes: -it, -ip ,-in, -is. Although 'is' is a useful word, there are not many high frequency words that end with these letters. The rimes -it and -ip can be used with all the onsets so far presented.

1.   Print the letters *it* on a card.
2.   Take the rest of the consonants, and lay each one in turn next to the *it* ending. Say the beginning—then the ending—then blend them together to see if they make a meaningful word.

3. Look through the learner's reading book to see if they can find the letters *it* printed together. Sometimes it will say /it/, sometimes it will have a different sound (e.g. in 'write').
4. Play games (e.g. Pairs) where an onset and rime are printed on cards. Turn up one of each—if they make a real word, the player keeps the pair.
5. Play board games that require the player to complete words by adding an onset or a rime. This can be done verbally, or in writing.

As the learner progresses through the structure:

1. Use the wooden letters. Take out the relevant rime, and use the rest of the consonants to see if the result is a real word, or a syllable. Sometimes the resulting syllable might prompt a well known two-syllable word (e.g. mag: magnet).
2. Use the learner's reading book. Skim through, putting a pencil ring round every example of the rime. Then copy or write from memory every example recorded.
3. Using the word lists at the relevant stage of the structure, print the words in large, neat, well spaced letters. Remind the learner of the vowels. (Print them at the top of the page if you need to.) Ask the learner to put a dot under the vowel, and a ring round the vowel plus the rest of the word. The onset and rime will be visibly separated. The onset should be instantly recognized—it will be in the reading pack. Say the onset. Work out the rime—say the rime. Blend the two together to make a word (see p.148 for sample sheet).
4. Make Family Four games (see p.187), grouping the families according to the rime. Before using the rime for spelling, make sure that each of the letters has been presented for writing (p.96). The learner needs to know which letters are vowels. If necessary, write down the relevant vowels for the learner's reference.
5. Give the learner a 'spelling test'. Write down (or spell) the relevant rime. Then dictate a list of words with that rime. Ask the learner to break the word into two bits, saying the onset and rime separately, then writing the whole word. Then the learner can spell out loud the written word, using the names of the letters. As the learner progresses, it may be possible to spell the word before writing.

The dyslexic learner, perhaps with weakness in short-term memory, sequencing, and phonological processing, responds well to this approach. It is so much easier to handle two bits of information (cr-isp) than five (c-r-i-s-p). Seeing a group of letters associated into one sound unit is a foundation for use of analogy in reading, and use of sound patterns in spelling. Even quite sophisticated, elderly, intelligent learners get a kick out of scoring ten out of ten for a spelling test. If the task has felt like a hard one, the learner is not going to feel patronized just because the teacher thinks the spellings are easy!

Compound Words

In compound words, the units of sound are also the units of meaning. This makes them simple to divide into syllables in oral work (e.g. bathroom, anyone, cowboy, snowman). Looking at a compound word in print is more difficult. As one young learner, faced with 'The Elves and the Shoemaker' asked us, "How do you know where to put your thumb unless you can read the word already?" The learner needs experience in spotting the two units. Make games bringing together the two units (e.g. dominoes, pairs), and use shared reading sessions to draw attention to compound words.

Words with Suffixes

Quick recognition of common suffixes ('-ing', '-ed', '-er' and '-s') can provide a key to reading many words in the simplest reading books.

In shared reading sessions, encourage analysis of a difficult word: "Try covering up the ending. Can you read it now?"

Scan through print, ringing the chosen letter cluster (e.g. -ing): "If you take the 'ing' away, do the rest of the letters still make a word?" Then write a list of all the identified words.

Syllable Division Patterns

A simple formula can make a confused string of letters into neat, accessible syllables, and encourage skilled use of the thumb! (see p.153 for a sample worksheet).

Print a regular, two syllable word. Put a 'v' over each vowel. Put a 'c' over the consonants between the two vowels. Divide between the two consonants. Say each syllable in turn. Say the whole word.

Once the learner can confidently read nonsense 'cvc' syllables, this works beautifully and often gives the learner confidence to try syllable division in shared reading.

For spelling, ask the learner to repeat the word in separate syllables. Look it up in a simple spelling dictionary (e.g. *Spell it Yourself*, Hawker, 1962). Notice anything odd about the word (e.g. unexpected vowels in unstressed syllables like 'petrol', 'velvet'; silent letters in words like 'listen', 'answer'). Cover, write, check; test again later in the session.

Advanced learners can be given the second most common syllable division pattern, found in words like *student*, or *pilot*. Put a 'v' over each vowel. (see p.179 for a sample worksheet). Put a 'c' over the consonant between. Divide after the first vowel. The first vowel will have its long sound (same as the name).

Following these two patterns, we begin to understand why 'hopping' has two middle consonants, and 'hoping' has only one.

Advanced learners will also want to use words with prefixes (e.g. ex-, con-, re-). Prefixes are rarely accented, so their vowel sound can be indistinct (e.g. 'describe', 'report'). A very useful little reference book with information and examples of word formation using prefixes and suffixes is the Cobuild English Guide 2, Word

Formation (Sinclair, 1991). It is intended for the use of learners of English as a foreign language, a rich source of useful materials for the learner with specific problems in literacy development.

Skilled readers have a wide variety of strategies at their fingertips; we want to make these strategies available to the learner with literacy difficulties. During shared reading sessions, the teacher will be there to orchestrate the appropriate use of the various techniques, till they become automatic for the learner.

Reading and Writing Sentences

When a new sound has been introduced, we like to practise it in words. It is a good idea to try these words out in sentences. Although we have strong reservations about the use of structured prose extracts, it is very helpful for the learner to carry through the learning into a small language sample. We have included a sentence or two on many of the pages of the last section. As you can see, they are inevitably stilted, and we present them for reading as a skills activity, or as a sort of puzzle. Their main use is as brief dictation exercises. Where there is little meaning, context can be added by verbal elaboration.

1.   Explain that a whole sentence will be dictated, so make sure there is a capital letter and a full stop. This is the least complicated way of defining a sentence; the teacher is giving regular examples. Sentence dictation is a good forum for the discussion of a variety of stops, so we include questions and exclamations.
2.   Remember that the learner may not have the short-term memory capacity to hold the whole sentence. You may need to read the whole sentence, then explain that you will dictate it in shorter sections.
3.   Say the sentence (or part of it) and ask the learner to repeat it.
4.   The learner writes the sentence in perfect joined writing—an excellent opportunity for handwriting practice.
5.   Mark the sentence. We give a tick for each word, a tick for capital letters, a tick for the full stop, an extra mark for a special target word. One of the authors has been known to give a tick for every letter approximately in the right place—one short sentence could clock up 30 marks or more!

Use of Games

In the step-by-step programme, we have described a variety of games. Naturally, our rules are not definitive, and should be changed according to the needs of the learners. There are some generalizations:
1.   Games should be fun.
2.   Keep the rules simple and fair.
3.   Involve skill as well as chance.

4.   Be sensitive to the emotional need of the learners—learning to win and lose is a serious part of any curriculum, and should not be brutal.

5.   Be clear about the aim of the game. If it is intended to be a learning game, is the learner using reading, spelling, or just pattern matching?

6.   To ensure multisensory learning, include verbal expression, insisting that the players 'talk through' their actions.

Planning a Lesson

Identification of specific literacy difficulties can sometimes lead to extra provision. The one-to-one sessions described below are an effective use of time. The assumption is that the learner is spending the rest of the time in a mainstream class or a large group, receiving a broad and appropriate curriculum. The skills sessions are intended to increase access to the mainstream curriculum. Do not assume that skills learned in an individual session will be carried through into real reading and writing tasks. All the helpers involved with a learner need to be made aware of the learner's progress through the programme, so that skills can be internalized and integrated into everyday learning. If class teachers are kept in touch with the programme, they can adjust their expectations, follow useful routines in providing support for writing tasks, and ensure that reading tasks are appropriate. If this sort of support within the classroom is not available, make sure that some of the sessions are devoted to planning, redrafting and presenting free writing. Don't assume that 'someone else' is responsible for the transfer of learning. A new piece of knowledge or a new skill is useless unless it has an aim and a purpose. Our hair stands on end at memories of learners given skills totally out of context; we remember Darren, a young Yorkshireman of 13, who was taught to fill in elaborate charts illustrating the spellings of long and short vowels, and the use of soft 'c' and 'g'. His younger brother showed him a card—"What does this say, Darren?"; "Nay, I don't know!". It said 'clock'!

'One-to-one' Skills Sessions

We acknowledge that 'one-to-one' teaching is not a magic formula that will solve all problems; the time has to be carefully and skilfully used, and appropriate methods employed. But many children have educational needs that are so specific and personal that it is difficult to see how they will make progress without some individual time. The programme does not always have to be delivered through a teacher; we have worked successfully with well trained and skilled special support assistants. The following activities form 40 to 50 minute sessions, and offer a good balance of skills training integrated into real reading and writing.

1.   Read a book (see p.61). Take a few minutes to enjoy rereading a book, easy enough to ensure success. The rest of the activities can be taken in any order, but a pleasant read is an essential beginning. Look at any completed homework.

2. Alphabet and dictionary work. Lay out the alphabet arc of wooden or plas-
    tic letters (see p.90). Games and activities to teach or reinforce knowledge of
    alphabetical order, letter name knowledge, sound–symbol links, word build-
    ing and analysis, short-term memory development.
3. Reading pack. Practise sounds so far covered (see p.102).
4. Spelling pack. Use the cards to practise the letter–sound links covered for
    writing (see p.102).
5. Introduce new work. Move through the structure (p.124), and work on a
    new sound–letter link, onset or rime for reading and writing.
6. Word reading and writing (p.102). Practise the new sound in words. Use
    lists, games, or scan through print.
7. Sentence reading and writing (p.110).
8. Introduce a new book (p.61). Check that the level is suitable by using a
    simple 'running record'. Notice strategies being used, and think about next
    goals. Use the book to notice and reinforce that day's new work.
9. Discuss homework, complete record sheets, sort out links with other teachers
    and parents—setting up effective channels of communication is essential.

Group Sessions

The reality of our teaching load does not always allow for working individually
with learners. Instead, we may spend much of our time working with small groups
or giving support within the classroom. The 'Skills into Action' programme can
be adapted for those of us who work in this way. Indeed, the broader aspects of the
programme can be applied to developing the skills of all learners, not just those
with special educational needs.

Example 1

All the group work together. The teacher directs and teaches the whole group,
helping individuals where necessary.

1. Individual rehearsal of the reading pack, and handwriting practice of letters
    and words covered so far.
2. Completed homework discussed and marked if appropriate.
3. Whole group revision of new work introduced last lesson, and assimilation of
    this into a reading and writing activity (e.g. work on building words using
    onset and rime; reading sentences containing the new letter sounds or words).
4. New learning. Introduction of a new letter sound, blend, or keyword.
5. Game to reinforce the new learning and to link it to more established
    knowledge.
6. Homework set (where appropriate).

Example 2

Teacher sets up a carousel of activities. The group members, working individually or in pairs, are directed through the series of tasks, receiving individual attention in turn.

1. Individual rehearsal of reading pack and handwriting practice of letters and words covered so far.
2. Completed homework discussed and marked if appropriate.
3. Carousel of activities
   (a) Alphabet activity.
   (b) Individual/shared reading.
   (c) Activity involving revision of work covered last lesson.
   (d) Game/computer activity to reinforce last lesson's work, or more established knowledge.
4. Whole group game reinforcing skills, or group reading.
5. Homework set (where appropriate).

Example 3

Whole group is focused on the same task, but work as individuals. Teacher facilitates discussion, helps learners begin, and leads the sharing of the work accomplished. Teacher circulates and helps individuals, highlighting teaching points for individuals and for the group as appropriate.

1. Individual rehearsal of reading pack and handwriting practice of letters and words covered so far.
2. Completed homework discussed and marked if appropriate.
3. Whole group discussion as a starting point for writing.
4. Individual planning/writing/redrafting.
5. Each learner shares work with the rest of the group.
6. Homework set (where appropriate).

An example of a lesson planning sheet is included (p.114). The sheet aims to act as an *aide-mémoire* for the different aspects of the teaching programme. It can be used for both one-to-one sessions and for groups. One sheet can be used for two or three letters to ensure that a variety of linked activities takes place. Areas causing concern, or progress made, can be recorded in the comments section with suggestions for the next lesson. The sheet can also be used to inform others involved with the learner about aspects of the teaching programme that have been covered. We regularly use this format for planning, and keep the sheets in a file alongside the learning objectives set for each learner (see p.60). Look at the examples of completed sheets (p.115, 116) to get a flavour of the way the proforma might be used.

Table 10.2 Lesson planning sheet

Name	Plan	Date Comments
Integrated reading/writing Shared reading Group reading Creative writing		
Alphabet Activities Visual Auditory Dictionary		
Sounds: Memory pack routines New card Onset and rime Words		
Writing skills New letter–sound Write on board Write on paper Onset and rime Words Sentences		
Word reading Keywords Regular words Target words		
Games/ worksheet		
Phonology Rhythm Rhyme Alliteration Syllables Onset and rime Phoneme		
Homework		

Table 10.3 Planning sheet		
Name *Jack*	Plan	Date *24.9.1995* Comments
Integrated reading/writing Shared reading Group reading Creative writing	*Read from current reading book. Encourage use of picture. Discuss before reading.*	*Jack looking at pictures more— using these with initial sounds when decoding.*
Alphabet Activities Visual Auditory Dictionary	*Lay out wooden letters in an arc. Say alternately with teacher.*	*Has to keep returning to 'a' to identify letters further on. Break alphabet into quarters to learn.*
Sounds: Memory pack routines New card Onset and rime Words	*Introduce 'a' to memory pack. 'at, ap, an' rimes for word building.*	*Good work. Next session work with 'it, ip, in' at same time for discrimination practice.*
Writing skills New letter–sound Write on board Write on paper Onset and rime Words Sentences	*Writing 'a' and three letter words with 'at, ap' and 'an' rimes. Sentence: 'It is a tap'.*	*Is stopping in the middle of words—try to encourage a continuous flow.*
Word reading Keywords Regular words Target words		
Games/ worksheet		
Phonology Rhythm Rhyme Alliteration Syllables Onset and rime Phoneme	*Auditory discrimination a/i*	*Further work on this needed—can do this from my speech but not from his own.*
Homework	*List of 'at, ap, an' words to learn for spelling.*	

Table 10.4 Planning sheet (group lesson)

Name *Year 10 group*	Plan	Date *28.11.96* Comments
Integrated reading/writing Shared reading Group reading Creative writing	*Read poem with '**qu**' words ('Rather him than me') as a group. Identify '**qu**'. Read sentence card with '**qu**' words in.*	*Jack and Ben read fluently. John and Kevin need more support. All identified '**qu**' words. Take poem home and reread next lesson.*
Alphabet Activities Visual Auditory Dictionary	*Lay out memory pack as alphabet. Note position of '**q**' and '**u**'.*	*John still reversing some letters but remembering order. Jack, Ben and Kevin can order alphabet unaided —try timing themselves next.*
Sounds: Memory pack routines New card Onset and rime Words	*Revise '**qu**'. Make '**qu**' words from pack (see words listed below).*	*Jack confusing '**i**' and '**e**'— include discrimination game next time.*
Writing skills New letter–sound Write on board Write on paper Onset and rime Words Sentences	*Write to dictation: 1.Dan put a quid in the tin. 2. Quick it's the Bill! 3. Tom had a pen in the quiz.*	*John needing lots of encouragement but can spell from teacher's exaggerated example. Kevin cannot hold whole sentence in memory. Jack and Ben forgot punctuation. Jack confusing **i/e**.*
Word reading Keywords Regular words Target words	*quick, quiz, quack, quid, quill, quit.*	*All able to decode through onset and rime.*
Games/ worksheet		
Phonology Rhythm Rhyme Alliteration Syllables Onset and rime Phoneme	*Look at the rhyming words within the poem—highlight and discuss.*	*Rhyming words identified.*
Homework	*Take home poem to discuss and read.*	

Homework is not always set, but frequently is! It may consist of any of the following:

1.   A piece of reading.
2.   Questions to answer on a passage read.
3.   Keywords to learn for reading/spelling.
4.   A section of the alphabet to learn.
5.   A worksheet to reinforce skills taught.
6.   A game to reinforce skills taught.

Older learners can be expected to complete tasks within their capacity without any help. Younger learners may need support and help from parents. If so, make sure that the tasks you set are appropriate and clearly explained. Check that they will not cause conflict between parent and child—some learners have undergone years of fruitless reading practice, soul-destroying for parent and child. Discuss the situation with the parents, and get a clear picture of what can be expected. Then make sure that homework tasks are very specific and limited. Say, 'Ask your Mum if she will help you prepare this poem for reading aloud to the group,' or 'Ask your Dad if he will help you practise this book so you can read it to your little sister'.

Liaison between the class teacher and the support teacher is essential. Their work must link together. The work within the support sessions should be relevant to the learning in the classroom, not isolated from it. It is crucial that the class teacher does not become disempowered by the support teacher's 'expertise', abdicating responsibility for the learner to the 'specialist' teacher. The support teacher also needs to spend time in the classroom to observe the learner and help with the transfer of new skills. When learners return to their classroom after a support lesson they can be encouraged to show their teacher their work, and to take part in reinforcement activities with peers, playing a game they have been given, or sharing their written work. (It is acknowledged that this is not always convenient.)

Part 3:
The Step-by-Step Programme

This section takes the teacher and learner step by step, page by page, through a series of sound–letter links. If the routines described in Part 2 are followed faithfully, and carefully adapted to individual needs, the learner should build automatic, speedy links, both for recognition and recall. Late readers are often poor at generalizing skills, and your learners will need help in moving an isolated bit of knowledge into memory banks so that it can be accessed to inform the whole language task of reading and writing. Look again at p.111 to see the make up of a lesson, and remember to constantly link the new letter sound into shared reading and writing sessions.

As each letter is introduced, materials are presented at different levels. The teacher will decide which level to choose. The learners must find the work challenging, but well within their capacity—success is vital. Success in learning is the basis of real, long-term gains in self-esteem. The teacher earns the learners' respect by guiding them through a fruitful learning process.

Sample worksheets and games are included, which can be adapted to the needs of the individual, and used at different stages of the programme.

Step-by-Step Programme

Presenting the programme

Pace

The pace depends on the circumstances. The age of the learners, the degree of disability, the time available, all affect the rate at which the programme is taught. In one school, young children with an average rate of learning, but with speech and language difficulties, will be steadily working through the programme, alongside their normal 'whole language' education, for four years. In another group, children in mainstream classes with mild dyslexic difficulties, cover at least one sound–symbol link every time they see their support teacher, and reach the end of the alphabet in 20 sessions or so.

Letter Order

This letter order was developed by the authors in response to the needs of the professionals and learners at the Rowan School, incorporating changes made on various courses taught for the Sheffield LEA and Sheffield University's Division of Education. Like Gillingham and Stillman (1969), Cox (1967) and Hickey (1977), we start with 'i, t, p, n, s'. Those five letters have many advantages. The 'i' and 't' are very distinctive letters, and easy to write and pronounce; together, they make a word. A large number of words can be generated from those letters, including consonant blends, and this gives a lot of freedom in producing early materials at different levels—the phonological development of the learner can be taken into account from the start. The letter order for children with spoken language difficulties should be worked out with a language therapist, starting off with sounds that the learner can make and recognize.

Clue Words

Where children are taught in groups, it is helpful to choose the same clue words so that they can learn from each other, and prompt each other. Our particular clue words were chosen because:

1.   They provide an example of a clear pronunciation of the sound in question. (/s/ in sun is clearer than /s/ in snake.)
2.   The words are the ones we come across in a child's environment.
3.   They are not likely to be confused with each other (avoid mouse /ow/ and rat /r/).
4.   They are as easy as possible to pronounce, bearing in mind the most likely problems of immature articulation.
5.   They are fairly easy to draw, and can be copied from our examples.

However, they do reflect the personal preference of the authors, and there is no reason why teachers should not choose their own clue words, as long as they follow the guidelines above. Trial and error soon reveal the snags.

The letter order sheets can be photocopied, and used as record sheets. Separate columns are provided to indicate when a sound has been taught for reading (R) or for spelling (S); teachers will adopt their own code to indicate mastery, and the level at which the sound is used.

We have included the most common rimes, and the ones that give a route to using analogy in word reading. As each new letter is introduced, the onsets already taught are repeated, and printed just above the newly available rimes. Use the letters and the lists of rimes to make real words and nonsense words. You can also print the rime onto a card, and use the onsets in the reading pack (see p.101). The word lists are not exhaustive. Our intention is to provide the teacher with enough sample words at each stage to provide an introduction to the word pattern for reading and spelling. In Section 1, Level 1 words have no consonant blends. Level 2 words have consonant blends at the beginning, at the end, or both. In Section 2, priority will be decided according to the learner's reading material and the words chosen for writing. In the interactive shared reading sessions, and in expressive writing sessions, attention will be drawn to patterns already covered— we hope, by the learner as well as the teacher.

We have also listed the keywords—these are the words taken from Cobuild's Bank of English (see p.105) and are the 100 most commonly used words. Each learner will also be collecting personal targetwords—family names, special interests, etc.

When teaching Section 1, it is important to maintain a very carefully structured approach. In the skills training part of the lesson, only include letters that have been covered. As the learner says the sound and writes the letter, links are being strengthened or even established, links that will underpin future development in reading and writing.

Section 2 has a suggested order, but at this stage teachers will be responding much more to the individual interests of the learner. The materials can still provide the basis for a systematic survey of sound–letter combinations, but the literacy programme can be built around the words that are encountered in everyday reading and writing tasks. If a particular sound is causing problems in a certain book, then teach it. The two examples here illustrate a less structured approach:

1. Simon is progressing through our programme, and is working at sorting out the choice for the /ā/ sound—'a-e' or 'ai'. He comes to a page in his Maths book which requires him to spell the numbers one to ten. He can spell them all except *eight*. His teacher follows the *Look—Say—Trace—Copy—Write* routine (see p.106). As part of the 'Look', the teacher gathers together all the meaningful words with the common 'eigh' grapheme (eight, eighty, eighteen, weight, freight, neigh, neighbour) and gives Simon practice in reading them.

2. Carol has completed the alphabet and can read and spell words with consonant digraphs 'th', 'sh' and 'ch'. She wants to use the word *characters* in her book review, but finds it confusing to write and to reread. She can already spell *school* correctly. Her teacher points this out, and writes a list of words, meaningful to Carol, where 'ch' has the /k/ sound, asking Carol to read the words and put a ring round the 'ch' (ache, Christmas, echo, character, chemist, orchestra, stomach).

Older dyslexic learners may benefit from a more detailed and extended structured approach (eg. Augur and Briggs 1992; Miles 1992). See p.218 for useful resources.

Letter order Section 1

front	back	R	S	useful rimes	keywords
i	igloo /ĭ/				I
t	tap /t/			it	it
p	pen /p/			ip	
n	nose /n/			in	in
s	sun /s/				is 's its
st	*stone /st/*				
sp	*spider /sp/*				
sn	*snail /sn/*				
a	apple /ă/			at ap an	a as at an
d	door /d/			id ad and	and said
h	house /h/				that his this has had than
e	egg /ĕ/			et en est ent end	the he she then
c	cup /k/				can
k	king /k/			ick ack eck	think
sk	*skip /sk/*			ask esk	
b	ball /b/			ab	be back been
r	ring /r/				are there her their
br	*bread /br/*				
cr	*cry /cr/*				
dr	*drum /dr/*				
pr	*present /pr/*				
tr	*tree /tr/*				
m	mouth /m/			im am amp	time them Mr
sm	*smarties /sm/*				him I'm me
y	yogurt /y/				by they my year years may says any
l	lolly /l/			all ell ill	all like last
bl	*blanket /bl/*				
cl	*cloud /cl/*				
pl	*plate /pl/*				
sl	*slide /sl/*				
f	fish /f/				if after first
fl	*flower /fl/*				
fr	*frog /fr/*				

Letter order Part 1 (contd)					
front	**back**	**R**	**S**	**useful rimes**	**keywords**
o	orange /ŏ/			ot op od ock ost	of to for on from not or one so no do some into only other also people most more
g gl gr	girl /g/ glove /gl/ grass /gr/			ag eg ig og	get
u	umbrella /ŭ/			un ug ut ub ull ump	but up about out could our because you your
j	jam /j/				just
v	van /v/				have over very
w	window /w/				was with we will which were who would now
sw tw	swim /sw/ twins /tw/				what when two new know
x	six /ks/			ax ex ix ox	
z	zebra /z/				
qu	queen /kw/				
th	thin /th/			ath	
sh	shop /sh/			ash ish ush	
ch	chips /ch/			atch itch unch	
wh	wheel /w/				
ng nk	sting /ng/ sink /nk/			ang ing ong ung ank ink unk	

Letter order Section 2

front	back	R	S
er	ladder /er/		
y (v)	penny /ĭ/		
	fly /ī/		
ee	feet /ē/		
ay	play /ā/		
oo	moon /o͞o/		
	book /o͝o/		
i-e	bike /ī/		
a-e	cake /ā/		
o-e	bone /ō/		
ea	beak /ē/		
	head /ĕ/		
ai	rain /ā/		
oa	soap /ō/		
ed	printed /ed/		
	pulled /d/		
	walked /t/		
u-e	tune /ū/		

front	back	R	S
ar	star /ar/		
or	fork /or/		
ou	mouse /ow/		
ow	snow /ō/		
	cow /ow/		
ce	space /s/		
ge	cage /j/		
ir	bird /er/		
ur	nurse /er/		
igh	light /ī/		
oi	point /oy/		
au	sauce /or/		
aw	straw /or/		
ie	thief /ē/		
ph	phone /f/		
ch	chemist /k/		
tion	station /sh'n/		
sion	mansion /sh'n/		

i

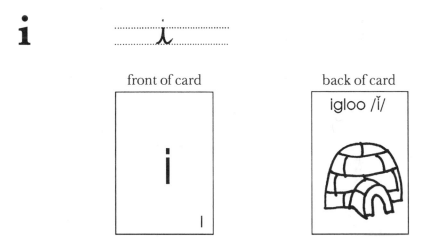

front of card — back of card

igloo /ĭ/

Listen: (see p.96) Colour the picture if there is an /ĭ/ in the middle.

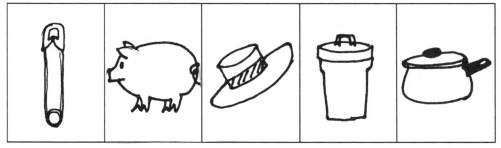

Look: (see p.96) Put a ring round every letter 'i'

i   I   i   I   L   T   i   t   T

Write and Say (see p.96)

Notice that the letter stays in the middle zone, except for the dot. Notice that the approach stroke is an inclined curve, and the letter 'i' drops straight down almost to the line before it turns up again. You need a leaving stroke to make sure that the next letter is suitably spaced. Teach the upper case from when you teach the keyword.

The teacher can write the letter 'i' in the learner's book, and establish the routine:

Trace, copy, write three times; tick the best.

Keyword: I

To write this keyword, the learner will need to be introduced to the capital form. As a general rule, we print the capitals, then start the rest of the word at the base line.

t

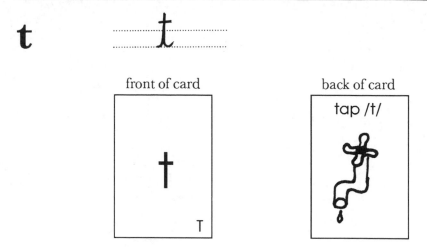

front of card   back of card

Listen: Where can you hear the /t/ sound; beginning, middle or end?

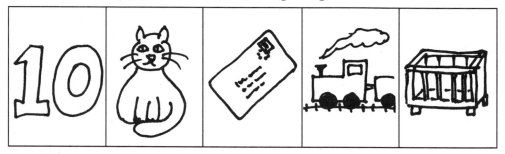

Look: Put a ring round every letter 't'

t   t   l   L   T   D   t   k   **T**   d

Write and Say

Notice that it goes into the upper zone. Its sound is unvoiced, and can be heard most purely at the ends of words (e.g. hit, pat, cat). Don't say 'ter'.

Using an exercise book with guidelines, let the learner trace, copy three times, and tick the best.

The capital has been included, but need not be taught for writing at this stage. The learner will need it for reading, as it will certainly be found in print—remember, the upper case print form is found on the front of each card.

Keyword: it

Let the learner write the word 'it', doing the whole word before adding the dot and cross. Think of more words that end in 'it'. Look for the two letters together in a current reading book—notice the sound they make.

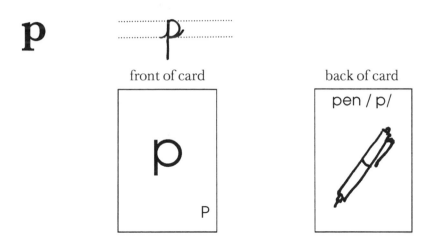

front of card   back of card

Listen: Ask the learner to listen to these words, repeat each one, and decide where the /p/ sound is heard: beginning, middle or end?

pin, pet, tap, happy, stopping, prize

Look: In a magazine or newspaper find and highlight some different forms of the letter 'p'.

Write and Say

Teach the letter 'p' for writing. Notice that it goes into the lower zone. Its sound is unvoiced, and can be heard most purely at the ends of words (e.g. stop, cap, step) . Don't say 'per'.

Word Writing Routine

If necessary, the learner can begin by making the word using the letters laid out in an arc. Then physically divide the onset from the rime (p-it, t-ip). Say the two bits separately. Put the letters back in the arc, and write the word down. Then spell the word, looking at the letters. Spelling means naming the letters—for younger learners, we say 'use grown up spelling' We are making a start in the establishment of a simple routine:

Listen—repeat—sound out—spell—write.

Words for writing

tip pip pit

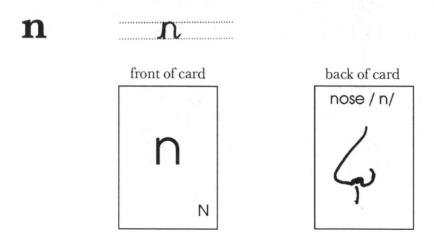

front of card   back of card

Using the ideas on the earlier pages, *Listen, Look, Write and Say.*
Notice that the letter 'n' stays in the middle zone. Make sure that the 'stick' does
not extend into the upper zone—if it does, it looks like an 'h'. When you say /n/,
the air goes down the nose—you can't say it properly if you have a bad cold!

Keyword: in

Write the words 'nip', 'in' and 'pin'.

Word Building, Using Onset and Rime Cards (see p.107)

Write the rime 'in' on a different coloured card next to the left hand edge. Explain
that 'in' can be a word, or the ending of another word. Take the memory pack,
and put the vowel aside—what you have left are onsets. Try each consonant in
turn, blending the onset and rime together, and see if they make a real word. With
'nin', the learner has been given the relatively painless experience of reading a
nonsense syllable.

*This technique can be used at every stage of the structure. The more frequent rimes are listed in the
letter order lists and in the word list tables.*

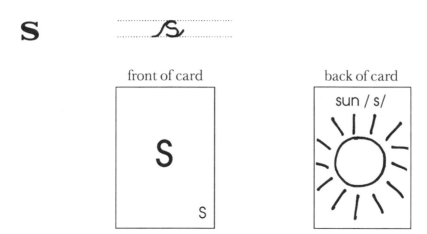

front of card

back of card

sun / s/

Listen, Look, Write and Say

Notice that the letter 's' can have a voiced or unvoiced sound—compare its sound in 'is' and 'this'. Feel the vibrations in the throat.

Help the learner to keep the letter in the middle zone. Write a few examples with mistakes, including some that are too tall, and ask the learner how they could be improved—it's more fun to criticize the teacher's efforts!

We normally teach each capital letter as it is needed to start a sentence or a name, but teaching the capital 's' now can help a learner to distinguish between upper and lower case. A simple print capital is easiest, although some teachers will prefer to teach the cursive form.

Onsets: t p n s (plus st, sp, sn if these sounds have been introduced)

rimes	level 1	keywords
in		is in
it	sit	's
ip	sip	its

If the learner can remember new sounds fairly quickly, and is very confident in saying the reading pack, give the blend cards 'st' and 'sp' ('sn' is possible at this stage, but not very useful). Examples of the pictures are given on p.174. It may be that the learner will find them helpful in reading—readers respond strongly to initial sounds and blends, and they can give a quick key to a word in a text. It might be some time before the learner can manage them for writing.

At this stage, you could explain that 'it's' and 'isn't' are contractions; 'it is', 'it has' and 'is not' are written as one word, without a space. The apostrophe marks the letter that has been omitted. You might also look for the possessive 's in a reading book–don't worry about it for writing, but it will be useful for reading.

In a shared reading session, you may find that a learner can read a singular noun but can't manage the plural (e.g. cat, cats). Try reading games matching pictures and words. The learner has to match a single object with the singular word, and more than one with the plural. Point out that the plural 's' is always just added—we need no apostrophe.

a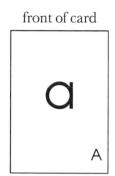

front of card   back of card

apple /ă/

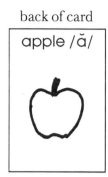

A

Use a vowel card—the same colour as the 'i'.

Listen, Look, Write and Say

Look in a mirror and notice the shape of the mouth when you say /ă/.

The letter stays in the middle zone. Make sure that the downward and leaving stroke are sensed as two movements—learners often dash off the last bit in one careless curve. Encourage the learner to stay in control until the end of the letter.

Southern English speakers will need to add another sound and picture on the card—say apple /ă/, glass /ah/.

Onsets: t p n s

rimes	level 1	level 2	keywords
at	pan	snap	a
ap	tan	spat	
an	nap	past	as
	tap	ant	at
		pant	an

Try writing a simple sentence or two. Use only the sounds taught so far for writing. Because the language will inevitably be stilted, use your imagination and your spoken language skill to give a credible context.

First *look* at the sentence. Read it. Notice that the sentence starts with a capital letter, and ends with a full stop. Practise the keyword, especially if it is irregular. Some learners will need to practise each word, making them one by one with the wooden letters. After writing, give a tick for each word, and extra ticks for punctuation.

Sentences: (a) It is a tap.   (b) Tip it in a pan.

By now the routines for rehearsing the memory packs should be well established: (see p.102).

Reading

Look at the front of the card. *Say* the clue word, then the sound.
Check by looking at the picture.

Spelling

Listen to the sound. *Repeat* it. *Spell* (name the letter/s). *Write.*

Sample worksheet Auditory discrimination of /ĭ/ and /ă/

What to do: Put a blue counter on 'a' words. Put a yellow counter on 'i' words.

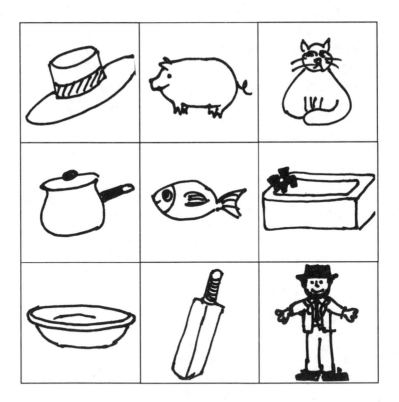

d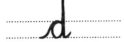

	front of card		back of card	

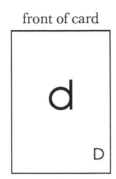 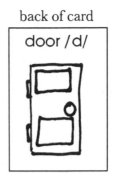

Listen, Look, Write and Say

Give this letter a careful multisensory introduction. Look in a mirror—see how the lips are apart and pushed slightly forward. Draw the letter in the air, using big arm movements, and link with the sound and name. Master the 'eyes shut' stage (see p.99). Notice that the letter is very like the 'a', but goes into the upper zone. Remember to stay in control until the end of the letter—the leaving stroke is important in determining the distance between the letters. Remember to use all the space in the middle zone.

Unless the learner mentions it, don't refer to b/d confusion—it is best to teach each letter separately.

Onsets: t p n s d

rimes	level 1	level 2	keyword
id	dip		said
ad	did	sand	and
and	sad	stand	
	pad		

level 1: (a) Dad is sad. (b) Dip it in a pan.

level 2: (a) Stan is past it. (b) Stand in a sand pit.

Learning Irregular Words

Read pages 105 and 106 for details of a routine for learning words that we find useful.

The 'S.O.S' routine (Simultaneous Oral Spelling) is described by Bryant and Bradley (1985) in *Children's Reading Problems*. It is particularly effective when learners have mastered letter names. The learner looks at the word, says it, then traces it, naming each letter while writing.

Hickey's routine (Augur and Briggs, 1992) is similar to the 'S.O.S'. The teacher writes the word in joined handwriting, on the blackboard or on paper. The learner looks at the word, says it, then traces it, naming each letter while writing. When the learner is ready, the word is copied, then written from memory, then written with eyes shut.

Once a word has been learned, check regularly until it is being written automatically in free writing.

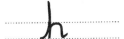

h

front of card

back of card

house /h/

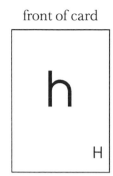

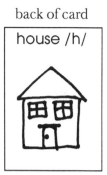

Listen, Look, Write and Say

Place the letter carefully in the correct zones—only the 'stick' rises through into the upper zone, and should be tall enough to avoid confusion with the 'n'.

Say /h/, not /her/—it's just a breath. Feel it on your hand. Some learners don't use this sound in normal speech; you might have to treat the letter 'h' like a silent letter (e.g. 'k' in knife, knee) finding ways of remembering its presence even if it is not articulated.

level 1	level 2	keywords
hat	hand	that
hip	hint	his
hid		this
hit		has
		had
		than

The irregular words become regular once the 'th' sound has been introduced. At this stage, the learner will need to approach the word as a whole irregular word.

level 1   (a) Pat hit Sid.   (b) I hid in a tip.

level 2   (a) An ant is in this tin.   (b) This is his hand.

e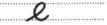

| | front of card | | back of card |
| | | | |

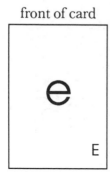

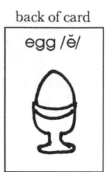

(use a vowel card)

Listen, Look, Write and Say

This is the only approach stroke that cuts diagonally across the letter. Keep in the middle zone.

/ă/, /ĕ/, and /ĭ/ can be easily confused—look in a mirror and see how the shape of the mouth changes as you say each sound.

Onsets: t p n s d h

rimes	level 1	level 2		keywords
et	ten	sent	nest	the
en	pen	tent	pest	
est	hen	dent	test	he
ent	net	spent	send	she
end	pet	step	spend	then
	set			

level 1   (a) Ted is ten.   (b) The hen is a pet.

level 2   (a) She is a pest.   (b) He set Ned a test.

Ladder Game: Vowel Discrimination

These ladders can be used for a variety of purposes. This one is used to encourage sound discrimination.

The game is for three players and a caller. Copy the ladders and stick them on separate cards, one for each player. Cut 21 small cards, one word on each (e.g., nip, pin, sip, dip, did, sad, pad, Dad, ten, pen, hen, net, pet, cat, bad, bet, bin, man, men, dim). Put the little cards face down on the table, or in a bag. Say, 'These words will have the sound /ă/, /ĕ/ or /ĭ/ in the middle. Listen for your own sound. You can move your counter up the ladder each time you hear your sound'. The caller takes a card and reads it. The first to reach the finish is the winner.

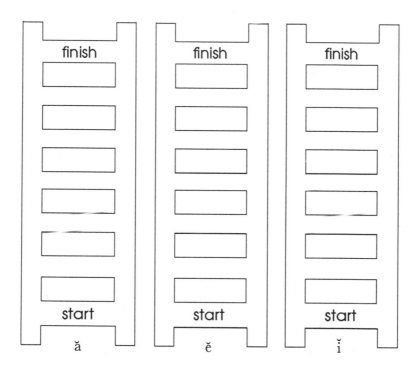

C

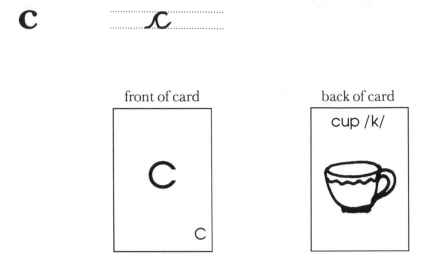

front of card   back of card

cup /k/

Listen, Look, Write and Say

The sound symbol could be /c/ or /k/; the latter is more consistent as it always says /k/, and the letter 'c' can be pronounced as /s/ in words like *city* or *dance*.

Keep the letter in the middle zone. Make sure the learner can remember the letter name.

level 1	level 2	keyword
cat	act	can
cap	tact	
	pact	
	cast	
	scan	

level 1   (a) Ed has a cap.   (b) Is the cat a pet?

level 2   'I can act,' said Ted.

The speech marks can be taught for writing, or just noticed for reading. Don't forget to base this work in real reading and writing—look for speech marks in various texts; notice the use of the comma at the end of the speech. Use speech 'bubbles' to give practice in writing speech. (see p.76).

k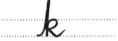

front of card   back of card

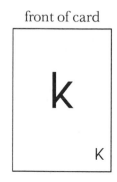   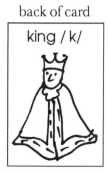

Listen, Look, Write and Say

This is a difficult letter to write. Notice how only the 'stick' rises into the upper zone. Make sure that the name can be spoken clearly and without hesitation.

Onsets: t p n s d h k (avoid 'c' before 'e')

rimes	level 1	level 2	keyword
ick	kid	ask	think
ack	kit	task	
eck	Ken	desk	
ask	Kit-kat	skid	
esk		skin	
		skip	

level 1   (a) Ken has his kit.   (b) He has a pet kid.

level 2   (a) Pat can skip.   (b) The pen is in the desk.

This is a good point to offer the learner the concept of a spelling choice. The sound is /k/, and there are different ways of spelling it. The rule varies according to derivation or position within a word—don't offer too much confusing information; deal with the rule a bit at a time, playing games to exercise and consolidate each stage.

From now on, when you practise the sound spelling routine, you will need to specify the context of the sound. So say 'How do you spell the /k/ sound in 'cat'? in 'king'?'

Spelling choice for /k/

Spelling rule: At the beginning of a word or syllable, the /k/ sound can be spelled with a 'c' or a 'k'.

First choice: 'c'. If the next sound is /e/ or /i/, choose 'k'.

Pairs (sometimes called Pelmanism) is a good game for practising spelling choices. Below are some pictures for you to use in making a pairs game. They all begin with the /k/ sound. Copy them twice onto small cards, making identical pairs. On the back of one of each pair, write the 'c' or the 'k', whichever represents the /k/ sound in that particular picture.

Lay out the cards, blank cards in one group and lettered cards in another, picture side down.

First player turns up a blank card and says the word represented by the picture. If the sound is /ki/ or /ke/, choose a card with 'k' on it. Anything else, choose a card with 'c' on it. The players MUST articulate their choice, naming the letter (e.g. 'I choose a 'c'' or 'I choose a 'k'') If there is a matching pair (e.g. two cats, or two kings), keep the pair and have just one more turn.

The winner is the one with the most pairs.

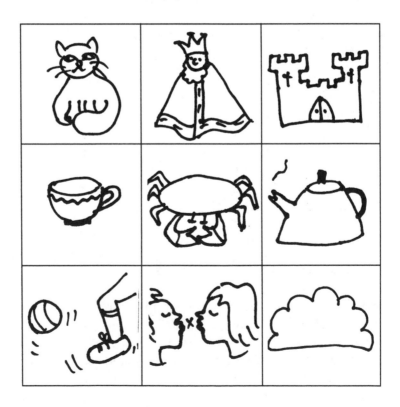

Spelling Rule

At the end of one-syllable words after one short vowel, use 'ck' for the /k/ sound.

Onset and Rime Activity

Make rime cards with 'ack', 'eck' and 'ick' on them. See how many real words you can make using your consonant cards (take the letter 'c' out of the pack unless you think the learner can already handle the soft 'c' rule). How many real words can you recognize? They should produce the following syllables. The words and non-words in brackets should be available for the learners who have the blend cards in their packs.

tack, pack, nack, sack, dack, hack, kack (+ stack, snack, spack, skack)
teck, peck, neck, seck, deck, heck, keck (+ steck, sneck, speck, skeck)
tick, pick, nick, sick, Dick, hick, kick (+ stick, snick, spick, skick)

If the learner recognizes *nack* as a word, you may decide to disallow it because the silent 'k' is missing—such rules depend on negotiation between the teacher and the learners. You have to decide between you if 'heck' is a word, or just a slang expletive. You have to decide if names (e.g. 'Dick') are going to be allowed.

This activity can become an independent writing exercise—ask the learner to make words with cards, and write out all the real words.

Pairs Game

Take 20 small cards. Write one word on each card, matched in pairs because their rimes are the same—draw attention to the rimes by writing in a different colour, or underlining. Lay the cards out in a grid formation, blank side up. In turn, the players pick up two cards, and read the words. If they have the same rime, they are kept as a pair. If successful, the player has one more go. The game moves along more quickly if some of the pairs are duplicated, and any of four cards could be used as pairs. Use any of the letters and rimes so far covered.

Suggested words: pip, tip, skip, nip, tap, snap, hat, pat, tick, sick, stick, kick, pack, tack, sack, snack, hack, neck, peck, deck.

Sentences for Reading and Writing

level 1   (a) Pat is sick.   (b) Pack the hat in a sack.

level 2   (a) Ted had a snack.   (b) The hen can peck the stick.

b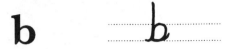

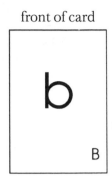

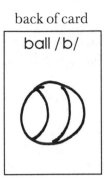

front of card   back of card

Listen, Look, Write and Say

Give a thorough multisensory introduction—the approach stroke to the letter 'b' should feel distinctly different from the approach stroke to the letter 'd'. Use a big arm movement. The circle should fill in the middle zone, touching the guideline.

Onsets: t p n s d h c b k

rime	level 1		level 2	keywords
ab	bad	bin	best	
	bat	ban	stab	be
	bed	Ben	bend	back
	bet	bit	bent	been

level 1   (a) The cat is bad.   (b) Ted is in bed.

level 2   (a) Ben's pen is bent.   (b) This is the best bat.

For some learners, a careful introduction to 'd' and 'b' is enough to disentangle the confusion. Most learners will need a bit more help—the important thing is that they have a method that they relate to, one that they feel responsible for.

Respond to the lip position—notice that when you are about to say the /b/ sound, your mouth is straight, in a line—write the line first. When you are about to say /d/, your lips are rounded—write the round bit first.

Remember a word, one that is never confused (e.g. 'and'), using it for reference.

Learners often have suggestions of their own—the most important thing is that they take responsibility for actively choosing and adopting a strategy.

r

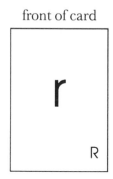

front of card

r

R

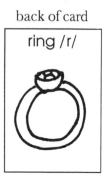

back of card

ring /r/

Listen, Look, Write and Say

This letter leaves from the top—pay special attention to its links with other letters. Explain that you have to get from the end of the 'r' to the start of the next letter, but need to approach on a slight upward curve.

level 1	level 2		keywords
rat	rest	trip	are
ran	drip	trap	
rap	brick	rent	there
red	crab	track	her
rid	dress	trick	their
rip	press	crack	
rack	cress		

level 1   (a) His kit is red.   (b) The rat ran in.

level 2   (a) That tap drips.   (b) Rick and Ben are here.

Introduce the 'r' blend cards when appropriate (see p.174). Don't teach them too quickly. As a rule of thumb, we prefer to keep the pack at a level where the learner forgets a maximum of three cards. Prioritize blends that might be causing problems in a current reading book.

Press, dress and *cress* should not present a problem for reading. Introduce them for writing when the learner needs any of them in writing activities.

m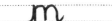

front of card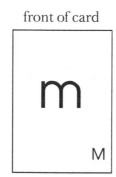

back of card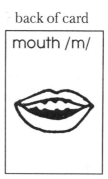

Listen, Look, Write and Say

Say 'mmm' not 'mer'. Notice how the air comes down the nose, and the lips are shut. The letter stays in the middle zone.

Onsets: t p n s d h c k b r ('r' blends as appropriate)

rimes	level 1		level 2		keywords
im	am	mad	camp	mask	time
am	ham	man	damp	mint	them
amp	him	map	tramp	trim	Mr
	dim	men	stamp	tram	him
	Tim	mass	cramp	pram	I'm
	met		mast	smack	me
	miss		mend	Mick	

level 1   (a) The man is mad.   (b) The ham is bad.

level 2   (a) This camp is damp.   (b) Mick can mend the map.

miss and *mass* for reading only.

Word analysis, using onset and rime

During shared reading sessions, learners may demonstrate a poor ability to 'sound out' even simple, regular short vowel words. The following technique may increase this skill .

1. Write the word on a piece of paper.
2. Identify the vowel, and put a dot under it (or a 'v' over it).
3. Put a ring round the ending, including the vowel.
4. Cover the rime; say the onset. Cover the onset; say the rime.
5. Say each bit in turn. Say the whole word.

Sample worksheets (level 1 or level 2)

Put a 'v' over the vowel. Put a ring round the vowel and the ending. Read the word. (vowels: 'a', 'e' and 'i'). The first one is done for you.

măn	cap
pan	tap
sat	tip
hat	dip

mĕnd	smack
bend	track
send	camp
spend	stamp

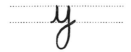

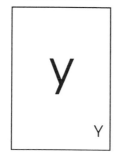 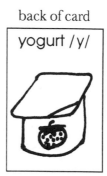

front of card   back of card

Listen, Look, Write and Say

This is the first letter with a looped leaving stroke. Teachers who are working with a learner withdrawn from a mainstream classroom may need to check that this will cause no problems—see p.96 to remind you of the forceful arguments for adopting a fluent cursive letter formation.

Older learners are often interested in graphology—the idea that some people will write whole books about letter formation, assuming that lower loops have significant things to say about the writer's emotional and social being, is fascinating to them. It can help them take a keen interest in the shapes they are making.

level 1	level 2	keywords	
yes	yank	by	says
yap	yell	they	any
yet		my	may
		year	
		years	

level 1   (a) Sit by me.   (b) It is my bed.

level 2   (a) Dad says yes.   (b) They can yell.

1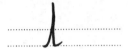

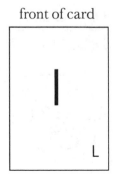

front of card

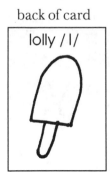

back of card

lolly / l /

L

Listen, Look, Write and Say

Say 'llll', not 'ler'. Notice that the letter goes into the upper zone.

Onsets: t p n s d c k h b r m y l (l blends as appropriate)

rimes	level 1		level 2		keywords
all	lip	lick	lend	smell	all
ell	lap	sell	list	spell	like
ill	lid	tell	lent	plan	last
	lad	ill	milk	plant	
	led	pill	silk	blend	
	let	bill	still	black	
	Len		spill	blast	

level 1 (a) Len bit his lip.   (b) Let Pam sit.

level 2 (a) Bill can spell.   (b) I can smell the bad milk.

Sample worksheet using onset and rime skills

What to do: Match the beginnings and endings to make real words. Write the words in the columns. Guess which column will have the most words.

t p n s d h c k b r m y l

(If appropriate: st sp sn sm tr pr cr br dr sl cl bl)

-all	-ell	-ill

f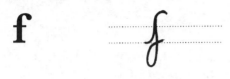

<table>
<tr><td align="center">front of card</td><td align="center">back of card</td></tr>
</table>

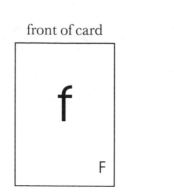

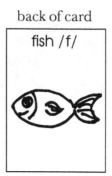

fish /f/

Listen, Look, Write and Say

This is the only letter that fills all three zones. The two essential elements are the hooked top, and the cross stroke. Make sure its 'back' stays straight—this letter can wobble about all over the place. Say 'fff' not 'fer'

If you like, you can introduce the f-blends—/fr/ and /fl/ (see p.174).

level 1		level 2		keywords
fat	fell		fast	if
fit	fill		fist	after
fin		daft	lift	first
fan		flat	staff	
fed			cliff	

level 1 (a) Deb fed the cat.   (b) The ham is fat.

level 2 (a) Fred's hen is daft.   (b) The flat has a lift.

Syllable Division

Give experience of dividing two-syllable words in oral work (see p.78). The following example worksheet uses a simplified version of Hickey's syllable division routine. The integrated approach to reading presents this as one possible technique for attacking longer words in shared reading sessions. At first it is mechanical and slow, but it becomes automatic.

Syllable Division: VC/CV Pattern

You may need to use the onset and rime division for reading each syllable (see p. 148).

1. Put a 'v' over each vowel.
2. Put a 'c' over the consonants between the two vowels.
3. Draw a line between the two consonants.
4. Read the word, then use the word in a sentence.

vc/cv pic/nic	kidnap	blanket
rabbit	kitten	absent
ticket	admit	bandit
dentist	intend	distant

O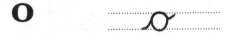

front of card	back of card

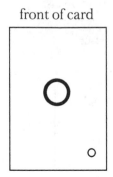

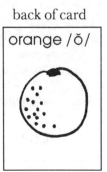

orange /ŏ/

Listen, Look, Write and Say

This letter, like 'r', leaves from the top. Pay special attention joining it to other letters. Notice the slight dip of the leaving stroke—this is essential if the next letter is to be approached from below.

Onsets: t p n s d h c k b r m l f

rimes	level 1	level 2	keywords	
ot	dot	lost	of	no
op	hot	cost	to	do
od	lot	soft	for	some
ock	hop	spot	on	into
ost	sock	clock	from	only
	lock	block	not	other
	dock	pond	or	also
	rod	cross	one	people
	nod	from	so	most
				more

level 1   (a) The pan is hot.   (b) Tom can hop.

level 2   (a) His clock is lost.   (b) It cost a lot.

Internalizing 'Spelling language'

Most good spellers subvocalize the syllables of a longer word, stressing them equally so that each vowel gets its true value—we sometimes describe it to learners as saying the word like a robot might (hos- pit- al, con- tin- ent, pet- rol).

Say the word, then repeat it in separate syllables. Tap each one out as you say it. Place a counter on the table for each one.

Find the word in a dictionary (see p.92). Look at it carefully. Is there anything unusual about that word? Is there anything that will require a special effort to make sure you remember it?

Close the dictionary, and write the word, saying the syllables as you write it. Have it tested again later in the session.

This approach is not usually suitable for young learners—the words are being chosen to give practice in skills, and are more likely to be in the mental lexicon of older struggling readers. But it does provide good exercises in:

1.   Awareness of syllables.
2.   Phoneme segmentation.
3.   Sound awareness within blends.
4.   Sound modification (e.g. bad min ton).
5.   Use of alphabetical order.

This paves the way for genuine dictionary use, when the learner will be using the dictionary to find spellings or pronunciations.

We will list longer words that provide useful practice in use of dictionary and in sound–letter links. These following ones are useable when you have introduced 'o':

Longer words: petrol combat contact continent hospital
badminton confident criminal domestic optimist

g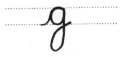

front of card	back of card
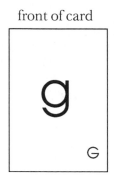	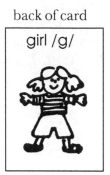

Listen, Look, Write and Say

Learners often find the name 'g' difficult to remember—use the *repeat- spell- write* routine. Some learners might still need to repeat, sound into onset and rime or phonemes, write, and then spell, looking at the letters they have written.

Onsets: t p n s d h c k b r m y l f g

rimes	level 1		level 2		keyword
ag	big	got	drag	grin	get
eg	dig	rag	flag	grip	
ig	pig	bag	frog	glad	
og	dog	gag	flog	grill	
	bog	leg	grass	gift	
	log	beg	glass	golf	
	gas	gap	grab		

longer words: magnet goblet goblin segment dragon glisten magnetic.

level 1   (a) Get the big bag.   (b) The pig is big and fat.

level 2   (a) The dog can dig in the sand.   (b) Get a grip on the bag.

Sample worksheet—Word search (Use words with common rimes)

What to do: Put a ring round the words (only across and down—not slanting).
Then write the words. Read them. What do you notice about them?

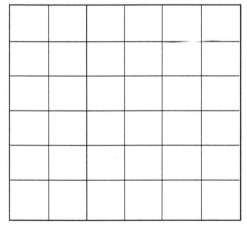

b	f	g	a	p	d
l	i	p	h	i	r
c	s	m	a	p	k
t	i	p	n	s	b
a	d	h	r	a	p
p	k	b	n	i	p

(answers)

b	f	g	a	p	d
l	i	p	h	i	r
c	s	m	a	p	k
t	i	p	n	s	b
a	d	h	r	a	p
p	k	b	n	i	p

Word search

Blank grid

Learners can devise similar word searches for others. Give a blank grid and a list
of words. Advise the learner to insert the words first, then add in the random
letters. They can use upper or lower case, but must print neatly. They can even
generate their own words—give a target rime (or two), and an onset and rime
sheet with the appropriate sounds printed on it (see p.151).

u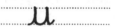

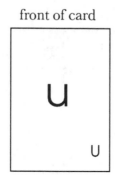

front of card

back of card

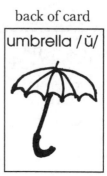

umbrella / ŭ/

Listen, Look, Write and Say

Northern learners have the same sound for /ŭ/ in bull and but.
Speakers of southern English will pronounce the two vowels differently. Point out that put and but do not rhyme, and draw attention to the sound of bull, pull and full. Link the 'ull' rime with 'ill', 'ell' and 'all'.

Onsets: t p n s d h c k b r m y l f g

rimes	level 1			level 2		keywords
un	put	fun	rug	dust	plump	but you
ug	cut	rub	dug	must	duck	up your
ut	nut	tub	full	rust	suck	about
ub	hut	mug	pull	dump	luck	out
ull	mud	bug	bull	bump	cluck	could
ump	bun	hug	cup	lump	truck	our
				pump	stuck	because

longer words: trumpet humbug sunlit muslin bullet crumpet disgust asparagus conduct.

level 1   (a) Get a big bun.   (b) Rob has cut his leg.

level 2   (a) Gus has a mug   (b) The hen is stuck in the mud.
                       of milk.

Suffix 'ed'

The suffix 'ed' is part of everyday language for young children. One of the first signs of awareness of syntax comes when they make up words using grammatical rules wrongly (e.g. 'I goed with Daddy'). Words with the 'ed' suffix are found in very early readers. For example, Oxford Reading Tree stage 3 *Roy and the Budgie*, uses the following words:

> jumped, locked, liked, looked, dropped, picked. (sounds like /t/)
> pulled, called, played. (sounds like /d/)
> wanted. (sounds like /ed/).

They demonstrate the three pronunciations of this suffix: /t/, /d/ and /ed/. The last pronunciation, where the suffix gives an extra syllable, is the least common.

If a learner can't read an 'ed' word, suggest covering the 'ed', and seeing if the rest of the word can be sounded out or recognized. For spelling, the learner may need a more conscious understanding of the rules that are being applied. In the early stages, it might be better just to tell the learner when a consonant is doubled or an 'e' is dropped.

Sample worksheet

What to do: Read* the poem. Put a ring round every 'ed' word. Write the 'ed' words in the boxes.

A Baby's Life

Baby played with his toes, and looked at his toys,
Kicked his legs in the air, and pulled the cat's tail,
Baby shouted for Mummy, then drank all his milk,
Hush! Baby is asleep.

played play + ed				

* The poem may be too difficult for independent reading. If so, read it to the learner, or read it together. You can make similar worksheets using reading material that is appropriate to your learner's interests and ability—for example, a sheet from a current reading book.

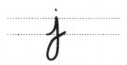

front of card	back of card
	jam / j / 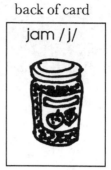

Listen, Look, Write and Say

Check that the written forms of 'f' and 'j' are not going to be confused—only the dot should be in the upper zone, whereas the 'f' should be as tall as a 'k'. Make sure that the letter name is being said very clearly—look in a mirror, and exaggerate the mouth movements for the names 'g' (jee) and 'j' (jay).

level 1	level 2	keyword
jam	jump	just
jet	jest	
job	junk	
jog	Jack	
jug		
Jim		

level 1   (a) Jim is on the jet.   (b) The man has a gun.

level 2   (a) Put the milk in   (b) This is just junk.
                      the jug.

Word Bases

Draw attention to the base 'ject'. Try to think of some of the words that come from this base, e.g. abject, object, subject, reject, project.

V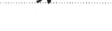

front of card

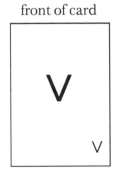

V

V

back of card

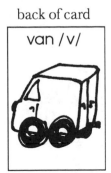

van /v/

Listen, Look, Write and Say

The sound /v/ feels the same in the mouth as /f/—notice the different feel in the throat. Cued articulation (p.37) makes demonstration of this very vivid. The written form can present problems—the rounded form is more harmonious, but can be confused with the letter 'u'. Make sure that the letter leaves from the top. Practise the 've' joining—some very common words end in 've'.

Spelling Rule

A simple rule, you will agree,
No English word can end in 'v'.

level 1	level 2	keywords
van	vest	have
vet	vent	over
vat	Vic	very
vim	vast	

Longer words: velvet invent invented invest investment.

level 1   (a) The big van is red.   (b) Vic ran to get the vet.

level 2   (a) Put a vest on.   (b) I have got a job.

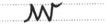

front of card	back of card
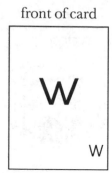	window /w/ 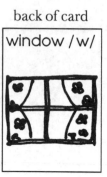

Listen, Look, Write and Say

Its form should resemble the 'v', but some learners who prefer the rounded 'v' still seem to prefer the pointed 'w', and it can take a lot of time for some learners to master the rounded one and still leave from the top. You may find that you have to compromise and have one rounded, one pointed—it doesn't really matter. You can add the consonant blends 'tw' and 'sw' if you think it is appropriate.

level 1	level 2	keywords	
wet	west	was	would
wag	twig	with	now
web	twin	we	what
win	went	will	when
wit	swim	which	two
well	swift	were	new
wig	twist	who	know
	swell		

Longer words: wigwam cobweb wedding twisted.

level 1 (a) I bet I will win. (b) The dog is wet.

level 2 (a) We can swim in the pond. (b) Pat went to get the twins.

X

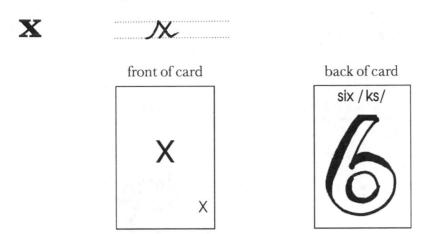

front of card   back of card

six / ks/

Listen, Look, Write and Say

All the cards so far have been vowels, or onsets. The letter 'x' is rarely used at the beginning of a word, and never with its most common sound /ks/. Learners find it difficult to say, unless they have been using cued articulation (see p.37)—making the two signs for /k/ and /s/ seems to make it clear. If it presents problems, leave it out of the pack, but give a full multisensory introduction to the rimes 'ix', 'ox', and 'ax'.

  This particular written form can be difficult to learn, but looks good when mastered. Show how it is approached from the bottom (mix) or from the top (box). Show how, like the letter 't', you need to go back and cross it.

Onsets: t p n s d h c k b r m y l f g j v w

rimes	level 1		level 2
ax	six	Max	next
ex	mix	box	text
ix	fix	fox	flex
ox	tax	sex	flax
	fax	vex	
	wax	Rex	

Longer words: index expect expel expand context.

level 1   (a) Rex is a big dog.   (b) Max has six pens.

level 2   (a) Send me a fax.   (b) Put the gift in a box.

Z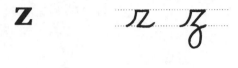

front of card   back of card

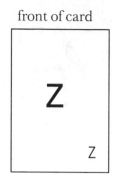   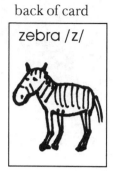

Listen, Look, Write and Say

The cursive form looks a bit eccentric, although learners usually seem to like it.
Decide between you which to adopt.

level 1	level 2
zip	zest
jazz	zinc
fizz	
buzz	

Longer words: zigzag zebra.

level 1   (a) Fix the zip.

level 2   (a) My zip is stuck.   (b) I listen to jazz.

Dictionary Work

   This is a good opportunity to focus on silent letters. Ask the learner to say
'listen', count the syllables, and isolate the first syllable. Look it up in a dictionary.
Ask the learner to look carefully, and see if they can notice anything odd or difficult to remember. Prompt if necessary until they have noticed the silent 't'.
Encourage its storage as lis-ten, emphasizing the /t/ sound. Let the learner close
the dictionary and write the word. Then go on to use it in a sentence.

qu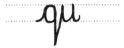

front of card

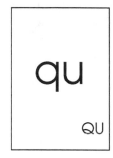

back of card

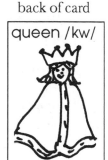

queen /kw/

Listen, Look, Write and Say

The letter 'q' is never used alone in English words, although it is often used at the end of commonly used names (e.g. Tariq, Iraq). Like 'z' and 'x', 'qu' is rarely used—none of the keywords have these letters in them. But ignorance of any letter can be confusing—it is important to complete the alphabet. Make sure the routines for introducing a new sound are faithfully observed—the learner will need help in mastering the articulation of sound, then letter names.

level 1		level 2
quit	quack	squid
quid	quip	squint
quick	quiz	quest

Longer words: inquest conquest squirrel.

Sentences: (a) Lend me a quid. (b) Be quick! (c) The ducks quack.

Handwriting: Completion of Alphabet

Now the learner can write the whole alphabet—this can occasionally take the place of work with the wooden letters.

Stages along the way (saying the names while writing).
1. Using 'tramlines', trace over an alphabet written by the teacher.
2. Trace over an alphabet printed lightly, then fill in the approach and leaving strokes.
3. Write the whole alphabet, aiming for increase in speed without loss of quality.
4. Move from the book with tramlines to ordinary lined book—write alphabet.
5. Do some copywriting (e.g. a short poem).
6. Do some task in an ordinary lined book—keep the task simple to start with.
7. Discuss with other professionals the need for the learner to adopt this handwriting style as the normal method of written expression. For some time, the new handwriting style will demand concentration, and that will limit the ability to focus on difficult or creative writing tasks. The learner will produce content *or* handwriting of high quality, but, for a time, not both.

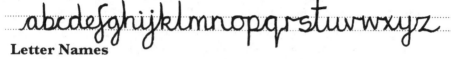

Letter Names

Don't forget to keep up the work on letter names. As your alphabet work includes more dictionary use, it is sometimes possible to forget that the learners may still need practice in setting out the alphabet letters in an arc, looking at, or listening to a sequence of letters, and taking them from the arc. Try also some 'feely' games:

1. Put some of the wooden letters in a bag, make sure you include 'j' and 'g'. Take it in turns to close the eyes, and draw out a letter, saying its name.
2. Put the two letters in front of the learner. Write one of them on the learner's back. The learner must point to the correct letter, and say its name. Vary the game by asking for name or sound. Let the learner take a turn at 'testing' the teacher.
3. Ask the learner to extend the writing arm, and to relax. You take the hand, and use it to 'write' a letter in the air, using a big movement. The learner will name the letter—make sure you include the difficult letters along with a selection of easy ones.

Ideas for Working with Suffixes

1. Photocopy a page from a suitable reading book. Ask the learner to scan each word, putting a ring round any word that ends in 'ed' (or 'ing', whichever is the focus of attention). Discuss the words together.
2. Use a page from a magazine or newspaper. Highlight any word ending in 'ed' (or 'ing'). Discuss the words together.

th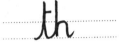

front of card	back of card

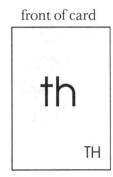

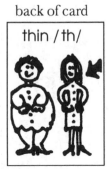

Listen, Look, Write and Say

Draw attention to the voiced and unvoiced sounds of 'th'. For reading, most learners who can sound out a word like with or this can make the modification from unvoiced to voiced without trouble. Sometimes they run into problems when they need the sound for invented spelling—you might like to add an example of the voiced 'th' onto the card. You can illustrate by using rebus symbols.

Onsets: t p n s d h c k b r m y l f g v w z qu th

rime	level 1		level 2
ath	bath	them	cloth
	path	than	thrill
	thin	this	fifth
	thick	with	sixth
	thud	that	tenth
	then		thump

Sentences   (a) The mud is thick.   (b) This bath is very hot.

(c) Ask them to go up the path.   (d) The box fell with a thump.

sh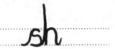

front of card	back of card

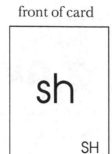

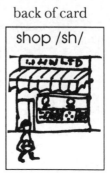

Listen, Look, Write and Say

Learners often confuse 'sh' and 'st' for writing—make a game (e.g. pairs or family three) that require their discrimination. Don't forget—the learners still need to *trace—copy—write from memory—write with eyes shut* saying the sound and repeating the letter names. Make sure the 's' stays within the middle zone. Make the card carefully to give a good example of the relationship between the letters.

Onsets: t p n s d h c k b r m y l f g j v w z qu th sh

rimes	level 1			level 2	
ash	shed	bush	dish		blush
ish	shall	push	fish		crush
ush	shock	rush	wish		shelf
	shut	ash		splash	shift
	shin	bash		smash	flesh
	ship	cash		clash	fresh
	shop	mash		crash	

Sentences: (a) The shop is shut.   (b) Put the fish on the dish.

(c) Vic lost all his cash in the crush.

(d) We will have to smash the lock.

ch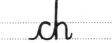

front of card	back of card

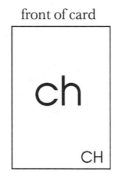

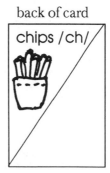

Listen, Look, Write and Say

Leave half the card blank. Another sound and picture will be added later (see p.215).

Most words that end in the /ch/ sound insert a 't'. You can offer a separate card with 'tch' on the front, and a clue word (e.g. match /ch/) on the back. Or you can present common rimes (e.g. 'atch', 'itch'), using them for reading games, and practising the handwriting patterns, linking them with the sound.

Onsets: t p n s d h c k b r m y l f g j v w z qu th sh ch

rimes	ch words			tch words
atch	chin	bench	patch	stitch
itch	chip	lunch	match	ditch
unch	chat	bunch	catch	switch
	chap	munch	batch	hutch
	chill	crunch	hatch	Dutch
	chop	punch	itch	much
	check	pinch	pitch	such
	chick	inch	witch	rich

Sentences: (a) Sam lit the match.

(b) The witch has a black hat.

wh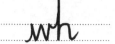

front of card

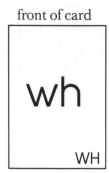

wh

WH

back of card

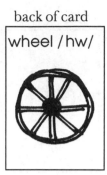

wheel / hw/

Listen, Look, Write and Say

Most young learners find it impossible to hear the difference between the first sound of *with* and the first sound of *wheel*. Neither do they pronounce them differently. You might find it easier to treat the 'h' as a 'silent letter', and give lots of games and activities to help the learner remember which are which. Most of the question words have the 'wh' start. Not many common words at this stage can be included, but you will find it useful when you reach the long vowels. Give special attention to the way 'w' and 'h' join together.

Ideas for Games: Pairs and Snap

1. Pairs. Make six pairs of cards, two each with the following words:

> when   which   where   why   who   what

Place the cards face down on the table. Players take turns in picking up two cards. If they get a pair and can read the word, they can keep them and have one more go.

2. Snap. Make a pack of about 30 cards. The words on them should begin with 'th', 'sh', 'ch' or 'wh'. Write the initial sound in a bright colour. The words do not have to be the same—the players can call snap for any matching initial blends.

Question Reading and Writing

This is a good time to revise question marks. Make cards with simple questions for the learners to read. Encourage them to make up questions for others to read and answer. They can be related to pictures from a magazine, or to a shared story.

ng

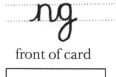

front of card

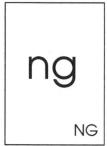

NG

back of card

sting /ng/

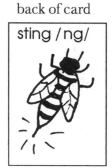

Listen, Look, Write and Say

This sound can be introduced after the letter 'g'. Without the support of cued articulation (p.37), learners find this sound very difficult to comprehend, isolate, and pronounce as a separate phoneme. You might prefer to ignore the card, and present 'ng' as part of a rime. 'ing' is the most useful, but there are also quite a few 'ang' and 'ong' words.

Onsets: t p n s d h c k b r m y l f g j v w z qu th sh

rimes	level 1			level 2	
ang	king	pang	rung	clang	spring
ing	ring	rang	dung	slang	bring
ong	sing	sang	lung	twang	fling
ung	wing	gang	hung	cling	strong
	bang	long	bung	sting	prong
	fang	song		string	stung
	hang	sung		thing	swung

Longer words: anything everything something.

Sentences: (a) Tom lost his ring.   (b) Liz can sing us a song.

(c) At last it is Spring!   (d) Bring me that thing.

Suffix 'ing'

The suffix 'ing' is found in easy readers with simple vocabulary, and can be quite confusing. In shared reading sessions, show the learner how to cover the 'ing' to make a difficult word become easy to recognize.

Sample worksheet

What to do: Read the word. Write it, adding 'ing'. Think of a sentence using the 'ing' word. Write it out, or dictate it to your teacher, then read it.

1. rush + ing
2. bang + ing
3. box + ing
4. miss + ing
5. bend + ing

Sample worksheet

What to do: Read the poem with your teacher. Put a ring round all the 'ing' words. Look at the first box—write out the 'ing' words like this.

Night	
Children dreaming,	Foxes hunting,
Mother resting,	Owls calling,
All in bed, sleeping,	Moon glowing,
The house is dark and still,	The night is alive.

dreaming
dream + ing

What to do next: Choose an article in a newspaper or a magazine, or photocopy a page of your reading book. Use a highlighter. See how many words ending in 'ing' you can find and mark in three minutes. Print them neatly in your book. Read them to your teacher.

nk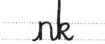

front of card

nk

NK

back of card

sink /nk/

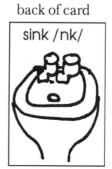

Listen, Look, Write and Say

Learners with good sound blending skills may be able to work out 'nk' words by saying /n/ /k/. Some learners may not be ready to learn 'nk' as a phoneme, and may need to work with the rimes 'ink', 'ank' and 'unk'.

Onsets: t p n s d h c k b r m y l f g j v w z qu th sh ch

rimes	level 1		level 2	
ank	ink	bank	thank	think
ink	link	sank	blank	blink
unk	mink	tank	clank	drink
	pink	Yank	plank	stink
	sink	bunk	spank	shrink
	rink	sunk	Frank	drunk
	wink	punk	swank	trunk

Sentences: (a) The ship sank.   (b) Put the dish in the sink.

(c) What do you think?   (d) I will have a drink of milk.

Pictures for Consonant Blend Cards

stone /st/ 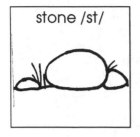	spider /sp/ 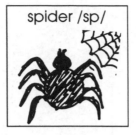	snail /sn/ 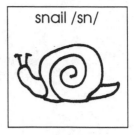
skip /sk/ 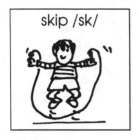	bread /br/ 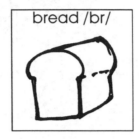	cry /cr/ 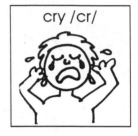
drum /dr/ 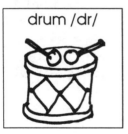	present /pr/ 	tree /tr/ 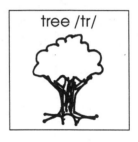
smarties /sm/ 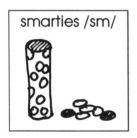	blanket /bl/ 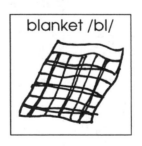	cloud /cl/ 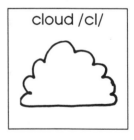
plate /pl/ 	slide /sl/ 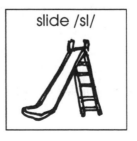	flower /fl/ 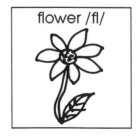

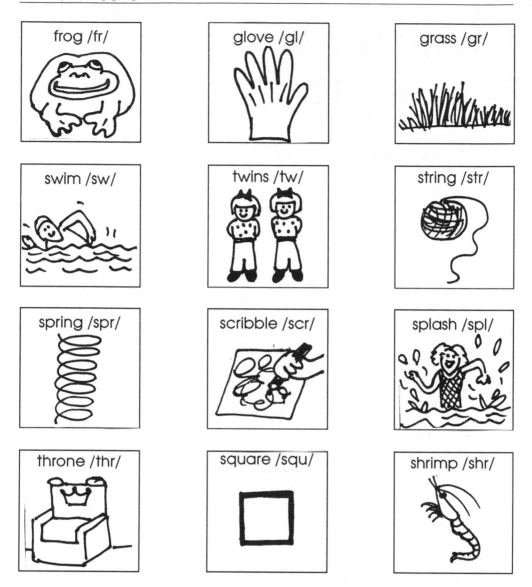

The reverse side of the consonant blend cards are shown here, with a picture to copy. Make the fronts as described on page 101—print the lower case in the middle of the card, and the upper case in the bottom right hand corner.

Chapter 12:
Moving Through
Section Two

Revision of Section 1

Before we begin work on Section two we want to be sure that the learner has become an accomplished user of alphabetic techniques. Can the learner:

1. Say the names of all the letters?
2. Link each letter with its most common sound?
3. Write each letter, lower and upper case?
4. Respond to initial sounds of words in shared reading sessions?
5. Use 'invented spelling' techniques?

Perhaps the learner has mastered the above at a very simple level, using only simple short vowel words with single consonats (cvc words) like *cat, pen, tin, pot, nut.* If so, it would be a good idea to see if the learner is ready to handle consonant blends. At this stage it is also useful to play lots of onset and rime games using all the alphabet. A useful source is the Phonological Awareness Training materials Wilson (1995) , which provide consolidation of alphabet knowledge and exercise of phonological skills for many of our learners.

Presenting Section 2

This section is less structured; we hope that by now the programme will be led more by the interests and needs of the individual learner. However, the principles of the programme are still the same. The aim is to build into the multisensory system automatic links between the letters and letter clusters *seen* by the learner, the sound they *hear*, the way it *feels* in the mouth and in the hand as it is written. It does not become a comprehensive, rule-driven spelling course. The word lists are not comprehensive—we aim to collect together enough useful words with a common sound pattern to provide material to work with. At this stage, the needs of the learner should be generating the material. The teacher will be responding to those needs that will emerge through shared reading and writing. At the same time, it is possible to take an active approach to skills acquisition, and to steadily build in knowledge of common letter clusters.

er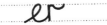

front of card	back of card
er ER	ladder /er/ 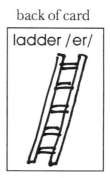

Listen, Look, Write and Say

The accented /er/ (as in 'stern') is unusual, but as an unaccented ending, gives a key to many common words.

(words with double consonants included for reading only)

ladder	number	finger	letter
tender	offer	winter	whisper
under	suffer	summer	jumper
thunder	dagger	hammer	temper
rubber	trigger	cracker	father
timber	stagger	better	mother
member	anger	sister	brother

Sentences: (a) I cut my finger.

(b) Listen to the thunder!

(c) The cat is under the bed.

(d) I am a member of the club.

When the letters 'er' are in an accented syllable, the pronunciation changes. Most of the words are not frequently used, but here is a list that might be useful:

her herd stern kerb jerk nerve swerve university deserve.

Adding suffixes 'er', 'est'

At this stage, you might like to introduce the suffix 'er'—it forms a comparative adjective (fast, faster) or suggests an occupation or pastime (painter, teacher). Choose vocabulary that is appropriate to your learner's needs. The sample worksheets give practice in using the suffix 'er' and 'est'. You don't have to use the complicated headings.

What to do: Fill in the boxes, adding the endings 'er' and 'est'. The first one has been done for you.

Adjective	Comparative	Superlative
fast	faster	fastest
thick		
old		
cold		
small		
black		

What to do next: Write three sentences, using these words:

1. thick 2. smaller 3. fastest.

Notice that only base words with double consonant endings have been chosen—it is never a good idea to introduce too many new ideas at one time. When you think the learner is ready, you can introduce the idea of doubling the final consonant of a short vowel, one syllable word ending in one consonant (e.g. *big bigger biggest*).

Spelling rule

A suffix can begin with a vowel or a consonant. If a suffix begins with a consonant (e.g. rest *ful*, hope *less*, dark *ness*) you *just add* it to the base word.

If your suffix begins with a vowel, you have to look at the ending of the base word. If it ends in two consonants, just add it. If it ends in one consonant, and has one short vowel, you *double* the final consonant.

big + er = bigger

Double Final Consonant of 'cvc' words

Sample worksheet

What to do: Add the ending. Double the final consonant. Write the new word in the box. The first two have been done for you.

fat + est	fattest	beg + ed	begged
thin + er		stop + ing	
fit + ed		clap + ed	
run + er		big + est	
win + er		put + ing	

What to do next: Read each new word in turn. Write (or dictate) a sentence using that word. Read it to your teacher.

Syllable Division: Long Vowel Pattern v/cv

Some common words ending in 'er' have a v/cv syllable division pattern. This might be a good time to introduce it. Here are some sample worksheets:

What to do : Put a 'v' over the vowels. Put a 'c' over the consonant between. Divide after the first vowel. It will have a long sound—the same as its name. Mark, then read to your teacher.

v / cv			
la /ter	baker	basin	bacon
safer	baker	later	Steven
evil	miner	Simon	driver
diver	glider	spider	robot
over	smoker	stupid	music

'le' Syllables

Another syllable division pattern applies to words ending in 'le'.

What to do : Put a ring round the last three letters. Read each syllable in turn. If the first syllable ends in a vowel, it will have its long sound.

-ble	-dle	-fle	-gle
table	candle	rifle	angle
stable	middle	trifle	single
bubble	puddle	raffle	jungle
bible	idle	snuffle	bugle
-kle	**-ple**	**-tle**	**-zle**
ankle	apple	little	puzzle
tickle	simple	battle	dazzle
buckle	maple	title	sizzle
crackle	dimple	cattle	guzzle

Use photocopied sheets or newspapers and highlighters to track and mark words with 'le' endings.

y

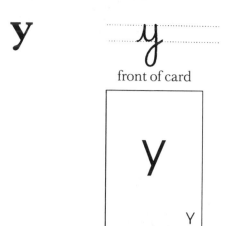

front of card

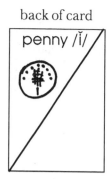

back of card

penny /ĭ/

Listen, Look, Write and Say

The learner will already have a white card with the letter 'y' on it. The clue word, *yogurt*, gives an example of 'y' as a consonant. Now the letter 'y' is being used to represent a vowel, so use a vowel card. Teachers often suggest that the sound at the end of 'penny' is /ē/ rather than /ĭ/. /ē/ is only heard in accented syllables. Say "jelly and custard", and you can hear the /ĭ/ sound.

A few words end in the letter 'i' -mini, taxi, bikini, corgi, and Italian pasta names (*spaghetti, ravioli* etc).

If the learner is not ready for the v/cv words, just introduce the ones needed for reading or writing.

vc/cv			v/cv
candy	penny	hobby	baby
handy	nappy	rugby	tiny
brandy	Daddy	empty	tidy
lorry	jelly	ugly	duty
silly	happy	Billy	lady
berry	Mummy	holly	crazy
carry	merry	plenty	ruby
nasty	pansy	dummy	lazy

Longer words: comedy everybody anybody somebody enemy agony hungry.

Sentences: vc/cv (a) The jug is empty.   (b) That was a nasty trick.

v/cv   (a) This is a tiny baby.   (b) I will tidy up.

y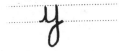

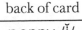

front of card   back of card

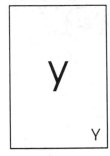   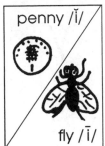

Listen, Look, Write and Say

Add the clue word *fly* onto the vowel 'y' card.
Ask the learner to make some of the words using the alphabet letters—you might find to start with you have to remove the letter 'I'—many learners will try to make 'MIY', 'BIY', etc.

my	try	fry	spy
by	cry	fly	shy
sky	dry	sly	why

Sentences: (a) My sister is shy.   (b) Andy can sit by me.

Suffixes 'y' and 'ly'

Older learners might find it useful to be introduced to these endings as suffixes. Add 'y' to a noun to form an adjective; add 'ly' to an adjective to form an adverb.

y			ly	
sandy	handy	fishy	sadly	richly
risky	rusty	filthy	gladly	sickly
windy	fluffy	rocky	snugly	thickly
bushy	tricky	chunky	strongly	dimly
milky	sticky	sulky	shyly	grimly
itchy	flashy	smelly	quickly	manly
messy	fussy	bumpy	badly	lastly

ee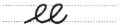

front of card	back of card
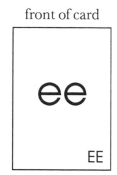	feet /ē/ 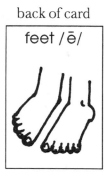

Listen, Look, Write and Say

This is the most common way of spelling the /ē/ sound in the middle and at the end of words—you can add a clue word for the end sound (e.g. three /ē/) if you like. Some of your learners may not be ready to isolate the /ē/ sound as a separate phoneme yet. You can use the words for onset and rime games.

deed	deep	cheek	been	see
feed	sheep	week	seem	bee
need	sleep	seek	feet	tree
bleed	peep	Greek	sleet	free
seed	cheep	feel	sheet	three
speed	keep	wheel	teeth	flee
greed	creep	steel	sweet	
weed	weep	seen	street	
green	sweep	meet		

Longer words: indeed chimpanzee canteen asleep sleepy
agree fifteen sixteen between.

Sentences: (a) The pond is deep.   (b) My cut began to bleed.
(c) Did you brush your teeth?
(d) She is fast asleep.

ay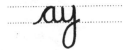

front of card   back of card

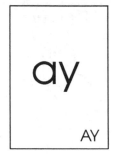

AY

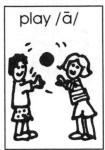

play /ā/

Listen, Look, Write and Say

bay	lay	ray	sway
clay	may	say	tray
day	pay	stay	way
gay	play	spray	slay
hay	pray	stray	

Longer words: away dismay decay delay holiday Sunday Monday Friday weekday yesterday display.

Sentences: (a) You stay here.   (b) It seems a long way.

(c) Put the glass on a tray.

(d) The stray cat was hungry.

Days of the week

At this point you might like to start teaching the sequence and the spellings of the days of the week. Be aware of the different techniques that will need to have been mastered by the learner. *Sunday* can be simply 'sounded out' by a learner who can manage two syllable words. *Friday* can be 'sounded out' by learners familiar with the long sound of vowels in v/cv words. *Monday* and *Wednesday* can be sounded out if the learner can modify vowels and store 'spelling language'. *Thursday* and *Saturday* will become transparent later on in the structure, when /ur/ has been introduced. *Tuesday* will always be an irregular word.

OO

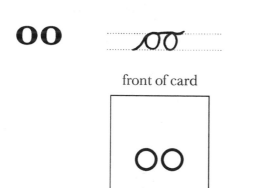

front of card

back of card

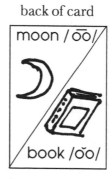

moon / ōō/

book /ŏŏ/

Listen, Look, Write and Say

You might want to introduce the two sounds on separate occasions.

When a learner is 'sounding out' a word, it doesn't matter which sound they start with—it is very easy to adapt from one pronunciation to the other. For writing, learners often use 'u' instead of 'oo' (e.g. *tuck* for *took* is a common mistake). We haven't found any helpful rules—just select from the array of whole word techniques (p.105-108, 136).

moon	cool	rool	book	hood
soon	fool	shoot	cook	stood
spoon	pool	zoo	hook	wood
noon	tool	too	look	blood
boom	stool		shook	
doom	boot		took	
room	hoot		foot	
gloom	loot		good	

Longer words: shampoo balloon foolish gloomy football understood mushroom bedroom baboon afternoon.

Sentences: (a) Get Jim a spoon.   (b) Roz likes cooking.

(c) Mr Smith is a good man. (d) Look at the moon!

i-e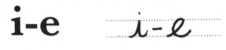

front of card   back of card

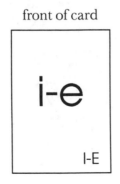

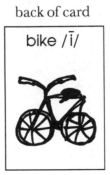

Listen, Look, Write and Say

Younger learners may find this card too difficult. If you are going to have to spend a great deal of time training the learner to respond to the card properly, then don't give it—older learners seem to cope with it so much more easily than younger ones, who can be given practice in reading and spelling the important words using onset and rime skills. This applies also to 'a-e' and 'o-e'.

ride	crime	line	while	bike
side	slime	bite	smile	like
wide	prime	kite	pile	pike
glide	chime	site	tile	spike
bride	mine	spire	stile	strike
pride	dine	quite	hire	rise
white	fine	mite	wire	wise
grime	shine	spite	spire	wife
mime	wine	file	drive	prize

Longer words: inside beside dislike reptile hostile textile vampire admire empire umpire invite.

Sentences: (a) It is a fine day.   (b) Nazim went on the slide.

(c) Have a glass of red wine.

(d) Rob took his Dad for a drive.

Vowel Consonant 'e' Words

Sample worksheet using onset and rime skills

What to do: Match the beginnings and endings to make real words. Write the words in the columns. Guess which column will have the most words.

b d f g h j k l m n p qu r s t v w sh th ch
(optional: gl sl br pr sp st sm gr)

-ime	-ile	-ine	-ite

Sample Game: Family Three

(Call it family four if you have four cards in each group) (two or three players)

Make nine sets of cards, one word on each: e.g. time, lime, chime; pile, tile, mile; mine, fine, line; bite, kite, quite; ride, side, hide; like, bike, hike; ripe, pipe, wipe; fire, wire, hire; dive, hive, drive.

Mark the rime by printing the common ending in a different colour.

Shuffle the cards well, and place them in a pile, face down.

First player takes a card and reads it, and places it face up on the table. The other player takes the next card and reads it. If it belongs to a different 'family' (i.e. it has the same rime) as the first card exposed, player two reads it and places it face up on the table. If it belongs to the same 'family', player two can take the first player's card, put them together and read them both.

Once the third card of a group has been collected, the 'family' is complete. The winner is the player with the most families.

a-e $a\text{-}e$

front of card   back of card

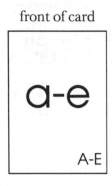

a-e

A-E

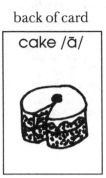

cake /ā/

Listen, Look, Write and Say

bake	drake	ale	ape	plate	plane
cake	take	blade	cape	came	mane
fake	whale	fade	shape	fame	pane
shake	dale	glade	rape	lame	shave
lake	gale	grade	tape	flame	brave
flake	pale	jade	date	frame	wave
make	sale	made	late	same	gave
rake	tale	shade	fate	tame	chase
brake	scale	spade	hate	cane	case

Longer words: cascade lemonade invade insane humane mistake.

Sentences: (a) We have the same name!

(b) You need a shave.

(c) The plane came in at runway three.

(d) Shall we sit in the shade?

o-e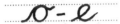

front of card	back of card

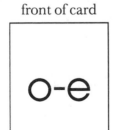

O-E

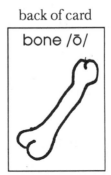

bone /ō/

Listen, Look, Write and Say

poke	dole	rope	shore	stone
choke	hole	Pope	score	zone
smoke	mole	slope	store	nose
bloke	pole	scope	cone	close
stoke	role	core	bone	rose
broke	sole	bore	drone	hose
stroke	vole	sore	throne	home

Odd words: one gone none done come some.

Longer words: tadpole maypole alone explore ignore impose expose primrose.

Sentences: (a) Shall we go home?

(b) I think my nose is too big.

(c) Don't smoke, it is a bad habit.

(d) The queen sat on the throne.

Adding Suffixes: Drop 'e'

If you add a suffix that starts with a vowel to a 'magic **e**' word, you have to drop the 'e'. You don't need it any more—the reader can see that the vowel stays long, because your new word ends having two syllables with the 'v/cv' pattern. (The 'ed' suffix does not always pronounce the extra syllable, but behaves as if it does, and the same rules apply as those that apply to 'ing' or 'est'.)

Spelling Rule

When you add a suffix starting with a vowel to a word with a 'magic e' (vce) ending, drop the 'e'.

Sample worksheets

What to do. Put a 'v' over each vowel. Put a 'c' over the consonant between. If you have a 'v/cv' word, mark the first vowel with the long vowel sound. Read the words to your teacher.

hoping	making	sloping	biting
baker	smoker	finer	wider
latest	finest	faded	safest

What to do: Read the word. Write the base word, then the suffix.
Don't forget to put back the dropped 'e'!

diving rider latest widest	dive + ing	hoping poking shining hated	hope + ing

ea *ea*

front of card	back of card

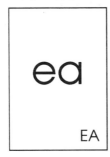

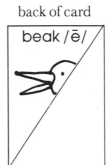

beak /ē/

Listen, Look, Write and Say

Leave half the card blank for the second sound (p.193).
If it is appropriate for your learners, present the spelling choice for the /e/ sound:
the most common way of writing the /e/ sound is 'ee'; this is a second choice, but
still important.

deal	beak	gleam	beat	bean
heal	leak	steam	cheat	clean
meal	peak	eat	each	mean
peal	weak	meat	peach	jeans
seal	speak	heat	reach	bead
steal	beam	neat	teach	lead
real	dream	seat	beach	read

You might also need the words ending in 'r'—this letter always alters the
pronunciation of the vowel.

ear fear gear hear near rear year

Longer words: repeat defeat.

Sentences: (a) You must speak to him.

(b) Jean won't eat meat.

(c) Play the game, but don't cheat.

(d) The children are on the beach.

Sample Game: Connect 4

You need two sets of counters—give one colour to one player, a different colour to the other. The first player puts a counter onto the board, first reading the word, then the second player does the same thing. The aim is to collect a row of four counters, down or across (diagonal is too complicated except for very able learners). If a player makes a mistake, they have to choose a different word.

beak	weak	speak	leak
eat	meat	seat	heat
neat	cheat	beat	mean
peach	reach	beach	clean
beam	dream	cream	teach
meal	heal	steal	deal

ea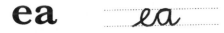

front of card	back of card
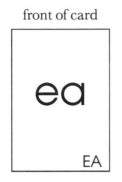	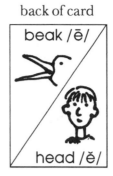

Listen, Look, Write and Say

Add the second sound onto the same card—the response will be 'beak, /ē/, head, /ĕ/'.

dead head read lead spread deaf heaven feather weather heather

Point out that *lead* can have the short or the long vowel sound, changing the meaning; with *read* the change in the vowel sound alters the tense.

This is an opportunity to introduce homophones—words that are spelled differently, have different meanings, but sound the same.

Spelling Choice 'ee', 'ea': Sample Worksheet

What to do: Look at the pairs of words at the beginning of each sentence. Choose one of them to fill the gap. Write out the whole sentence in your book (or write the word in the gap).

cheep cheap The dress is - - - - - . The chicken went - - - - - .	**been bean** Where have you - - - - ? I planted a - - - - .
heel heal Jane has a blister on her - - - - . This cut won't - - - - .	**steel steal** Someone will - - - - - it. It is made of - - - - - .
meet meat - - - - me at the bus stop. Dad will cook the - - - - .	**week weak** I am too - - - - to lift it. Seven days make a - - - - .

ai

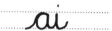

front of card

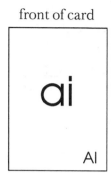

back of card

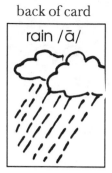

Listen, Look, Write and Say

This is the second choice for spelling the /ā/ sound. It is most commonly used before 'l', 'n' and 'r', but also used to distinguish homophones.

rain	sprain	sail	air	paint
pain	drain	pail	fair	faint
gain	grain	fail	hair	saint
brain	main	tail	stair	maid
plain	nail	jail	pair	paid
Spain	hail	mail	flair	wait

Longer words: contain obtain maintain .

Sentences: (a) Wait till it stops raining.

(b) I need a pair of socks.

(c) Jane has fair hair.

(d) The rain in Spain falls mainly on the plain.

oa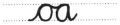

front of card

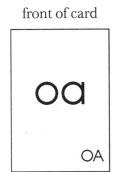

back of card

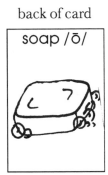

Listen, Look, Write and Say

Some learners find it really difficult to use these letter clusters as phonemes. You might find that they just keep forgetting the cards, however rigorously you follow the multisensory teaching techniques. If so, just take the card out of the pack and work on rimes (e.g. oak, oad)—either using a systematic approach, or responding to needs made apparent in shared reading or writing sessions.

oat	throat	soak	Joan	soap
boat	road	cloak	loan	oath
coat	load	croak	coal	boast
goat	toad	moan	goal	
float	oak	groan	foal	

Longer words: cloakroom oatmeal.

Sentences: (a) Joan likes that soap best.

(b) I live just along the road.

(c) Listen to that toad croaking.

(d) Edmund left his coat in the cloakroom.

ed

front of card	back of card
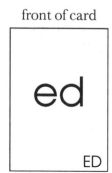	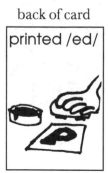

Listen, Look, Write and Say

Leave as much space as you can on the card for two other pictures (p.197).

In shared reading sessions, the learner will already have come across many words with this suffix. The teacher will have pointed out how difficult words are easier to recognize if you cover up the 'ed' ending, and used photocopies of shared texts for scanning exercises, putting a ring round every 'ed' ending. For spelling, the learner will have been taught that they need to think about action words ending in the /t/ or /d/ sound. Common invented spellings (e.g. *jumpt* and *kickt*) are incorrect, and must be examined carefully. For learners with poor cognitive skills or weakly developed phonological skills, you might prefer to maintain this approach.

Abler learners might find it helpful to know that the suffix 'ed' can be combined with the base forms of verbs to form the past tense (e.g. she *banged* the door, he *handed* me the book). It can also combine with nouns to form an adjective (e.g. a *gifted* child, a *hooded* coat).

mended	floated	killed	looked	passed
twisted	tinted	filled	booked	messed
handed	loaded	pulled	jumped	fussed
blended	lifted	yelled	bumped	pushed
landed	hooded	banged	walked	rushed
waited	gifted	clanged	talked	crashed

Longer words: adopted   invented   invested   intended   contented interested.

Sentences: (a) Tony has mended the bike.

(b) Mum has booked the holiday.

(c) We waited a long time for you.

(d) The van crashed into the wall.

When completed, the back of the card will look like this.

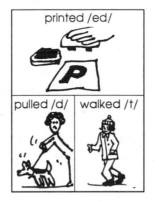

u-e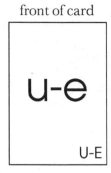

front of card	back of card

u-e

U-E

tune /ū/

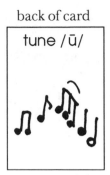

Listen, Look, Write and Say

There are so few words with this pattern that we rarely give this card. Depending on dialect, the pronunciation ranges between /ū/ and /ōo/. However, it is useful for a learner who appreciates patterns, and they might like to complete the group of all five long vowels. You might prefer to teach certain important words (e.g. use, June, cube) as they arise in real reading and writing.

cube	flute	fume	cure
tube	duke	fuse	pure
cute	Luke	use	sure
mute	June	mule	lure
lute	tune		

Longer words: endure compute confuse.

Also: picture nature puncture lecture capture mixture lecture adventure.

Sentences: (a) Luke can play the flute.   (b) The fuse has gone.

At the end of a word the /ū/ sound is quite rare—you might look at the two alternatives, 'ew' and 'ue'. Again, pronunciation varies.

new	threw	due	glue
few	knew	sue	true
chew	dew	hue	argue
grew	brew	cue	rescue
flew		blue	value

ar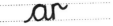

front of card	back of card

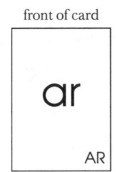 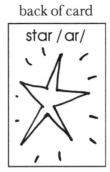

Listen, Look, Write and Say

The sound 'ar' is the same as the letter name, and this can cause confusion—young writers often assume that the single letter is enough for the whole syllable (R U my friend?). Pay close attention to the writing—make sure the stick of the 'a' drops down to the line before gently turning up again.

ark	spark	smart	lard	barn	bar
bark	shark	part	yard	darn	car
dark	art	tart	arm	yarn	far
lark	cart	start	farm	carve	star
mark	dart	card	harm	starve	jar
park	chart	hard	charm	Mars	scar

Longer words: carpet garden darling harvest discard regard alarm.

Sentences: (a) The children play in the park.

(b) Art is my best lesson.

(c) Henry is quite charming.

(d) A spark started the fire.

or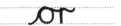

front of card

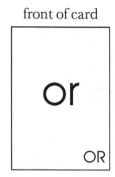

OR

back of card

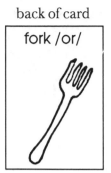

fork /or/

Listen, Look, Write and Say

Make sure that these letters are written clearly—there must be a distinct difference between 'or' and 'ar'. Their sounds are similar, and can look identical if written carelessly.

born	fort	fork	form	more	bore
corn	port	pork	storm	snore	core
torn	sort	stork	or	wore	store
horn	short	cork	for	sore	shore
thorn	sport	ford	horse	score	swore
scorn	snort	cord	gorse	tore	

Longer words: morning normal formal corner transform uniform.

Sentences: (a) Harry likes all sorts of sport.

(b) I like sweet corn.

(c) The horse has a thorn in its hoof.

(d) There was a bad storm this morning.

'wa', 'wo' words

Learners might like to observe the affect that the 'w' has on the following vowel sounds. Look in a mirror to see how much the lips have to move to change from /w/ to /a/. Many of the words are very familiar ones that will have already come up in reading and writing.

Useful words: was   wash   want   watch   wasp   swan   swap   war

warm   warn   swarm   word   world   worm   worst.

ou

front of card   back of card

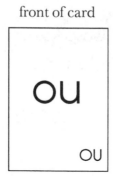   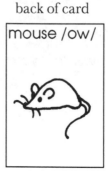

Listen, Look, Write and Say

This is a difficult sound—the mouth moves first into the position for the /ă/ sound. It needs a careful multisensory introduction, and lots of practice of the writing pattern.

round	ground	stout	mount	south
found	wound	trout	count	our
sound	out	scout	loud	sour
pound	bout	house	cloud	hour
mound	clout	mouse	proud	flour
hound	shout	louse	mouth	scour

Longer words: about aloud counter county rounders mountain fountain.

You might refer to some words with the same writing pattern but a different sound (your pour tour; four; colour flavour honour vapour favour).

Sentences: (a) Come and play in our house.

(b) We went South for four hours.

(c) Please don't shout.

(d) He is not fat, just a bit stout.

OW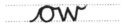

front of card

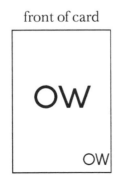

OW

OW

back of card

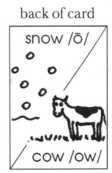

snow /ō/

cow /ow/

Listen, Look, Write and Say

Link the letters with both sounds in turn. Repeat, spell, write, first for the /ō/ sounds, then for the /ow/ sound. We would prefer to introduce the two sounds on separate sessions.

ow = /ō/		ow = /ow/		
bow	show	how	brow	gown
blow	slow	now	town	owl
snow	throw	cow	down	growl
grow	row	row	clown	
crow	low	vow	crown	
flow	glow	bow	brown	

Longer /ō/ words: window arrow borrow elbow shadow bungalow.

This is a good time to focus on silent letters—use the word *know* as an example. Discuss the problems of looking up such words in a dictionary. Include word on 'wr', 'kn' and 'gn'.

Longer /ow/ words: towel vowel tower shower bower.

Sentences: /ō/ (a) Show me your hands.

(b) The snow is quite deep.

(c) My plant is growing.

(d) Throw the ball to Janet.

/ow/   (a) The cow is eating the grass.

(b) The owl is hooting.

(c) Come down from that wall.

(d) That is Mark's towel.

Possessive 's is very common, and will have been encountered for reading—check that the learner can handle it for spelling.

ce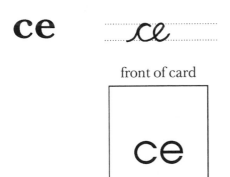

front of card

back of card

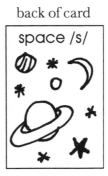

```
ce
                    CE
```

space /s/

Listen, Look, Write and Say

Younger learners will find it much more productive to learn important writing patterns (e.g. *ace, ice, ance*)—the idea of 'c' having the /s/ sound when followed by 'e', 'i' or 'y' is the sort of conditional rule that does not come easily to children under 9 or 10 years of age. It is a very consistent rule. The only exceptions are *soccer* and *sceptic* (*skeptic* in the USA). You can drill it into a bright child, but many learners will find it more productive to practise important writing patterns (e.g. *ace, ice*) and learn important words (e.g. *once*).

Older learners might like to look in a simple dictionary to see the words beginning with 'c', and pick out the important ones (e.g. city, centre, century, circle).

ace	place	glance	nice	mince
face	grace	prance	dice	since
lace	brace	France	spice	prince
pace	trace	chance	slice	wince
race	dance	ice	lice	
space	lance	mice	twice	

Longer words: romance entrance advance sentence absence December accident except.

Have a look at 'sc' words–scent, scissors, science.

Sentences: (a) This is a nice place.

(b) We will stay in France for a week.

(c) Grace ate her ice cream.

(d) I have been waiting since ten o'clock.

ge

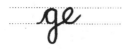

front of card

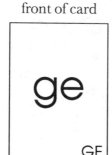

ge

GE

back of card

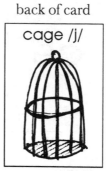

cage /j/

Listen, Look, Write and Say

Another conditional rule, with the same constraints as 'soft c'. 'Soft g' is less consistent—some very common words (e.g. *get, girl, give*) retain the hard /g/ sound. Again, you may prefer to use writing patterns of common rimes.

Draw the learners attention to the 'dge' pattern after a short vowel.

age	fringe	barge	ledge	fudge
cage	binge	charge	sledge	nudge
page	hinge	lunge	wedge	grudge
rage	tinge	gorge	bridge	
stage	winge	badge	ridge	
wage	large	edge	judge	

Extra words: change   exchange   danger   DANGER   stranger
damage   image   postage   luggage   village   baggage
cabbage   bandage   magic   imagine   giant   legend.

Sentences: (a) Don't go so close to the edge.

(b) This is a very large helping.

(c) Road rage is just bad temper.

(d) Jean's hamster has a nice cage.

ir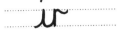

front of card | back of card

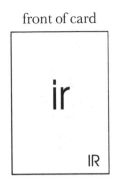

ir

IR

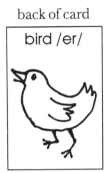

bird /er/

Listen, Look, Write and Say

When the letter 'r' follows a vowel, the resulting sound is always fairly indeterminate. The Scots differentiate between 'ir', 'er' and 'ur'; the English pronounce them all the same. Concentrate on words that are significant to the learner, and use the patterns of the rimes.

fir	lwirl	first	birch
sir	dirt	thirst	chirp
stir	shlrt	bird	firm
girl	skirt	third	
swirl	flirt	birth	

Longer words: thirty thirteen circle circus.

Sentences: (a) My hands are dirty.

(b) Betty's new skirt is torn.

(c) Karen came first in the race.

(d) Simon got a nice shirt for his birthday.

ur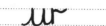

front of card	back of card

nurse /er/

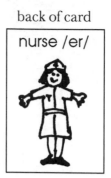

front of card box:

ur

UR

Listen, Look, Write and Say

fur	burn	hurl	purse
blur	turn	purl	curve
slur	churn	nurse	church
spur	curl	curse	lurch

Longer words: curtain murder surname Saturday surprise survive
Thursday murmur turban disturb.

Sentences: (a) Have you lost your purse?

(b) Mandy has a nasty burn on her leg.

(c) We will visit the church on Thursday.

(d) I wish my hair was curly.

igh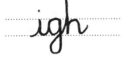

front of card	back of card
igh	light /ī/ 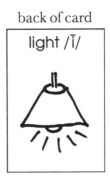
IGH	

Listen, Look, Write and Say

There are a few 'ite' words (see p.186), but 'ight' is more common. The fluent unbroken hand movement, including the looped 'g', is important for learners with sequencing problems.

bright	light	slight	thigh
fight	night	tight	nigh
fright	right	high	
flight	sight	sigh	

Longer words: delight alright fortnight.

Sentences: (a) Last night I had a bad dream.

(b) You gave me a fright!

(c) Turn the light off when you leave the room.

(d) Try not to get into a fight.

oi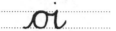

front of card   back of card

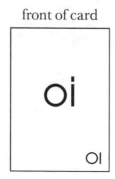   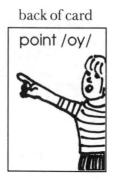

Listen, Look, Write and Say

oil	foil	groin	joint
boil	spoil	noise	joist
soil	coin	poise	hoist
coil	join	voice	
toil	loin	point	

Longer words: avoid rejoice.

Sentences: (a) It is rude to point.

(b) What's that noise?

(c) Put the pan on to boil.

(d) You need to put a pound coin in the slot.

Notice the 'oy' at the end of words: toy boy joy annoy employ.

au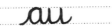

front of card

back of card

sauce /or/

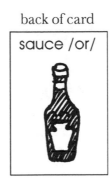

au

AU

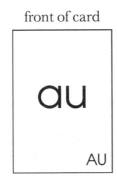

Listen, Look, Write and Say

Northern speakers say and hear *orb* and *daub* as rhymes. Southern speakers can hear a difference between the /or/ sound and the /au/ sound. They might like to use /aw/ for the sound symbol for 'au' and 'aw'.

haunt	clause	maul
gaunt	pause	launch
flaunt	gauze	cause
taunt	Paul	sauce
jaunt	haul	fault

Longer words: autumn   automatic   launder   laundry   saucer because.

Notice the common pattern (augh) in: caught taught daughter slaughter naughty

Sentences: (a) It is not my fault.

(b) Samantha ran from the haunted house.

(c) Paul puts too much tomato sauce on the pasta.

aw

front of card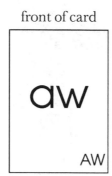

AW

back of card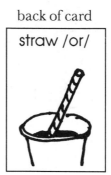

straw /or/

Listen, Look, Write and Say

saw	jaw	crawl	scrawl
draw	flaw	drawl	shawl
raw	law	brawl	lawn
claw	straw	trawl	dawn

Longer words: lawyer drawer hawthorn.

Sentences: (a) Paul hit Dave on the jaw.

(b) The lawn is full of weeds.

(c) Rose made a shawl for the baby.

ie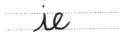

front of card   back of card

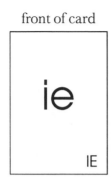   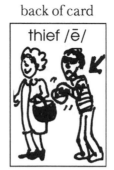

Listen, Look, Write and Say

thief	shield	piece
brief	wield	fiend
chief	yield	shriek
field	niece	priest

Longer words: mischief achieve believe.

Sentences: (a) The thief took the silver cups.

                (b) Have a piece of cake.

                (c) Piers is up to mischief.

                (d) The fiend gave a terrible shriek.

Most adults know one spelling rule: 'i before e except after c' . It is not a very meaningful rule for a learner who is struggling with the concept of spelling choice between 'ee' and 'ea', but might help sophisticated learners. The rule applies to *ceiling*, and to words derived from a Latin base meaning 'take' (deceit, deceive, receipt, receive, conceit, conceive).

ph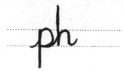

front of card	back of card

ph

PH

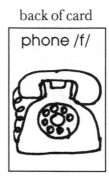

phone /f/

Listen, Look, Write and Say

phone	telephone	dolphin
graph	telegraph	elephant
photo	photograph	alphabet
orphan	orphanage	paragraph
nephew	phantom	physics

Sentences: (a) Philip is on the phone.

(b) I can say the whole alphabet.

ch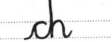

front of card   back of card

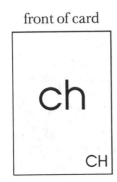   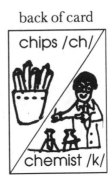

Listen, Look, Write and Say

The learner will already have a card with 'chips' /ch/. Add this new clue word to the /ch/ card.

chemist	orchid	chemical
school	orchestra	chemistry
echo	Christ	mechanic
ache	Christmas	technical
stomach	christen	character

Sentences: (a) Charles likes school.

(b) Chemistry is my best subject.

tion *tion*

front of card

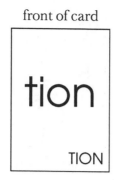

TION

back of card

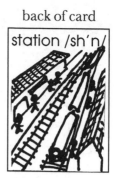

station /sh'n/

Listen, Look, Write and Say

You can treat this syllable like an 'le' syllable—put a ring round it, and then read the rest of the word. Or print it on a piece of card and let the learner cut off the syllable with a pair of scissors. Divide the rest of the word where it seems convenient, and be prepared to use trial and error.

action	motion	education
fraction	mention	information
section	addition	protection
nation	subtraction	multiplication
station	vacation	institution
lotion	perfection	expedition

Sentences: (a) The train is standing in the station.

(b) Don't mention it!

(c) I am looking for some information.

sion ‿‿‿sion‿‿‿

front of card

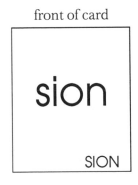

SION

back of card

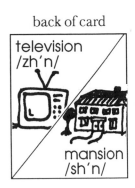

television
/zh'n/

mansion
/sh'n/

Listen, Look, Write and Say

vision	passion	pension
television	mission	emulsion
revision	admission	tension
division	expression	mansion
confusion	discussion	extension
explosion	procession	convulsion

Sentences: (a) I went to get my pension.

(b) The tension is mounting.

Another /sh'n/ ending is spelled 'cian'. Words ending in 'ic' (e.g. magic, physic, electric) take this ending: magician electrician musician physician mathematician.

Useful Resources

Books and Programmes for Teachers

Atkinson M. (1988) *Hear it, See it, Say it, Do it*, Cheerful Publications, 7, Oxley Close, Gidea Park , Romford, Essex RM2 6NX.

Augur J, Briggs S (Eds) (1992). *The Hickey Multisensory Language Course*, London: Whurr Publishers Ltd.

Clay MM (1975). *What did I write? Beginning Writing Behaviour*, Oxford: Heinemann Educational.

Clay MM (1993a). *An Observation Survey of Early Literacy Achievement*. Oxford: Heinemann.

Cooke A (1993). *Tackling Dyslexia the Bangor Way*, London: Whurr Publishers Ltd.

Hatcher PJ (1995). *Sound Linkages*, London: Whurr Publishers Ltd.

Hinson M, Gains C (1993). *A–Z Reading Books. A Graded List of Reading Books*, NASEN.

Hornsby B, Shear F (1980). *Alpha to Omega*, 3rd edn, Oxford: Heinemann Educational.

Miles E (1992). *The Bangor Dyslexia Teaching System*, London: Whurr Publishers Ltd.

Passy J (1993). *Cued Articulation*, Northumberland, UK: STASS Publications.

Reason R, Boote R (1994). *Helping Children with Reading and Spelling: A Special Needs Manual*, London and New York: Routledge.

Sinclair J (Ed.) (1991). *Word Formation*, Collins Cobuild English Guide, London: Harper Collins.

Stirling EG (1993). *Help for the Dyslexic Adolescent*, 8th edn, Published by St David's College, available from EG Stirling, 114 Westbourne Road, Sheffield S10 2QT, UK.

Stone C, Franks E, Nicholson M. (1995) *Beat Dyslexia!* LDA, Duke Street, Wisbech, Cambs. PE13 2AE.

Thomson ME, Watkins EJ (1990). *Dyslexia. A Teaching Handbook*, London: Whurr Publishers Ltd.

Van Oosteroom J, Devereux K (1992). *The Rebus Glossary*, LDA, Duke Street, Wisbech, Cambs PE13 2AE.

Walker J (1983). *Walker's Rhyming Dictionary of the English Language*, London: Routledge and Kegan Paul.

Wilson J (1995). *Phonological Awareness Training*, (Parts 1 and 2) available from Jo Barnard, County Psychological Service, 25 Buckingham Road, Aylesbury, Bucks HP19 3PT.

Useful Reading Schemes

Monster Books, Longman Education, Burnt Mill, Harlow, Essex CM20 2JE.

Oxford Reading Tree (compiled by Roderick Hunt), Oxford: Oxford University Press.

Rescue Readers, Trend, New Trend, Impact, (for older readers) Ginn, Prebendal House, Parsons Fee, Aylesbury, Bucks HP20 2QZ.

Spirals, (for older readers) Stanley Thornes, Ellenborough House, Wellington Street, Cheltenham, Glos. GL50 1YD.

Story Chest , One-to-one Stories , Trog books and *Wellington Square*, Surrey: Nelson.

Sunshine Books, Oxford: Heinemann Educational.

Ziggy Zoom Books, (from All Aboard Scheme) Ginn, Prebendal House, Parsons Fee, Aylesbury, Bucks HP20 2QZ.

Other Materials

Exercise books for handwriting, Cambridge Series, Ruling 9, *Philip and Tacey*, Northway, Andover, Hants SP10 5BA.

Hawker GT (1962). *Spell It Yourself*, Oxford: Oxford University Press.

Mackay D, Thompson B (1970, 1992). *Breakthrough to Literacy: Sentence Makers*, London: Longman Group, Burnt Mill, Harlow, Essex CM20 2JE.

Mosely D, Nicol C (1986). *The ACE (Aurally Coded English) Spelling Dictionary*, LDA.

Plastic letters (upper and lower case), Early Learning Centres.

Wooden letters (upper and lower case), Galt.

Assessment Material

Bradley L (1992). *Assessing Reading Difficulties*, Windsor: NFER-Nelson, (for a very informative Education Catalogue, Tel 01753 858961, Fax 01753 856830).

Graded Word Reading Test, Grades 6–12 (1985) Grades 9–14 (1990) The Macmillan Test Unit, Windsor: NFER-Nelson.

Hagley F (1987). *Suffolk Reading Test*, Windsor: NFER-Nelson.

Neale MD (1989). *Neale Analysis of Reading Ability*, British adaptation by Una Christophers and Chris Whetton, Windsor: NFER-Nelson

Peters ML, Smith B (1993). *Spelling in Context: Strategies for Teachers and Learners*, Windsor: NFER-Nelson.

Schonell FJ (1971). *Schonell's Word Reading Test*, Edinburgh: Oliver and Boyd.

Snowling MJ, Stothard S, McLean J (1996). *Graded Non-Word Reading Test*, Suffolk UK: Thames Valley Teat Co.

Vernon PE (1977). *Graded Word Spelling Test*, London: Hodder and Stoughton.

Vincent D, de la Mare M (1990). *Individual Reading Analysis*, Consultant Helen Arnold. Windsor: NFER-Nelson.

IT Resources

Crick Computing, *Clicker 2*, 123 The Drive, Northampton NN1 4SW, UK.

PAL (The Predictive Adaptive Lexicon), Scretlander Ltd, Glasgow

Phases, My World, SEMERC, 1 Broadbent Road, Watersheddings, Oldham, UK.

Writing Set, The Meldreth Picture, Symbol and Writing Suite, Widgit Software, 102 Radford Road, Leamington Spa, UK.

See also the *Computer-Users Bulletin* published by the Computer Resource group, British Dyslexia Association, BDA, 98 London Road, Reading, UK.

References

Adams MJ (1990). *Beginning to Read: Thinking and Learning About Print*, Cambridge, MA: MIT Press.

Adams MJ (1994). Learning to read: Modelling the reader versus modelling the learner. In: Hulme C, Snowling M (Eds), *Reading Development and Dyslexia*, London: Whurr Publishers Ltd.

Aitchison J (1987). *Words in the Mind. An Introduction to the Mental Lexicon*, Oxford, UK and Cambridge, USA: Blackwell Science.

Augarde P (1993). *Oxford Primary School Dictionary*, Oxford: Oxford University Press.

Augur J, Briggs S (1992). *The Hickey Multisensory Language Course*, London: Whurr Publishers Ltd.

Barr R (1974). The effect of instruction on pupil reading strategies. *Reading Research Quarterly* **10**: 555–582.

Bertelson P, de Gelder B (1989). Learning about reading from illiterates. In: Galaburda AM (Ed.), *From Reading to Neurons*, pp. 1–23. Cambridge, MA: MIT Press.

Bradley L (1980). *Assessing Reading Difficulties*, Windsor: NFER Nelson.

Bradley L, Bryant PE (1983). Categorising sounds and learning to read: a causal connection *Nature* **301**: 419–21.

Bruce DJ (1964). The analysis of word sounds. *British Journal of Educational Psychology* **34**: 158–70.

Bruck M, Treiman R (1992). Learning to pronounce words: the limitations of analogies. *Reading Research Quarterly* **27/4**: 375–388.

Bruner JS (1983). *Child's Talk: Learning to Use Language*, Oxford: Oxford University Press.

Bryant P, Bradley L (1985). *Children's Reading Problems*, Oxford: Basil Blackwell.

Burt C (1937). *The Backward Child*, London: University of London Press.

Burtis P, Bereiter C, Scardamalia M, Tetroe J (1983). The development of planning in writing. In: Kroll B, Wells G (Eds), *Explorations in the Development of Writing*, Chichester: John Wiley and Sons.

Carey S (1978).The child as word learner. In: Halle M, Bresnan J, Miller GA (Eds), *Linguistic Theory and Psychological Reality*, Cambridge, Mass.: MIT Press.

Chukovsky K (1963). *From Two to Five*, Berkeley and Los Angeles: University of California Press.

Clay MM (1972). *Sand—the Concepts About Print Test*, Aukland: Heinemann Publishers.

Clay MM (1975). *What Did I Write? Beginning Writing Behaviour*, Aukland: Heinemann Educational.

Clay MM (1979). *Stones—the Concepts About Print Test*, Aukland: Heinemann Publishers.

Clay MM (1993a). *An Observation Survey of Early Literacy Achievement*, Aukland: Heinemann.

Clay MM (1993b). *Reading Recovery: a Guidebook for Teachers in Training*, Aukland: Heinemann.

Collins Cobuild (1995). *The Bank of English*, London: Institute of Research and Development, Birmingham Research Park, Vincent Drive, Birmingham B15 2SQ.

Cooke A (1993). *Tackling Dyslexia the Bangor Way*, Birmingham: Whurr Publishers Ltd.

Cooke J, Williams D (1985). *Working with Children's Language Disorders*, Bicester: Winslow Press.

Cooper J, Moodley M, Reynell J (1978). *Helping Language Development*, London: Edward Arnold.

Cox AR (1967). *Structures and Techniques : Remedial Language Training*, Cambridge, MA: Educators Publishing Service Inc.

Crick Computing, *Clicker 2*, 123 The Drive, Northampton, UK.

DeFries JC (1991). Genetics and dyslexia: an overview. In: Snowling M, Thomson ME (Eds), *Dyslexia: Integrating Theory and Practice*, London: Whurr Publishers Ltd.

DFE (Department For Education) (1994). *Code of Practice on the Special Identification and Assessment of Special Educational Needs*. Crown Copyright.

Donaldson M (1978). *Children's Minds*, London: Fontana.

Dowker A (1989). Rhymes and alliteration in poems elicited from young children. *Journal of Child Language* **16**: 181–202.

Duane DD (1991). Neurobiological issues in dyslexia. In: Snowling M, Thomson ME (Eds), *Dyslexia: Integrating Theory and Practice*, London: Whurr Publishers Ltd.

Ehri LC (1995). Phases of development in learning to read words by sight. *Journal of Research in Reading* **18/2**: 116–125.

Ehri L C (1979) Linguistic Insight: Threshold of Reading Acquisition. In T G Waller and G E Mackinnon (eds) *Reading Research: Advances in theory and practice, Vol 1* 63-111. New York: Academic Press.

Ehri LC, Robbins C (1992). Beginners need some decoding skill to read words by analogy. *Reading Research Quarterly* **27/1**: 13–25.

Ellis AW (1984). *Reading Writing and Dyslexia: a Cognitive Analysis*, London and New Jersey: Lawrence Erlbaum Associates.

Fischer, FW, Shankweiler D, Liberman IY (1985). Spelling proficiency and sensitivity to word structure. *Journal of Memory and Language* **24**: 423–441.

Fox B, Routh DK (1983). Reading disability, phonemic analysis and dysphonetic spelling; a follow-up study. *Journal of Clinical Child Psychology* **12**: 28–32.

Frith U (1985). Beneath the surface of developmental dyslexia. In: Patterson KE, Marshall JC, Coltheart M (Eds), *Surface Dyslexia*, London: Routledge and Kegan Paul.

Frith U (1992). Cognitive development and cognitive deficit. *The Psychologist: Bulletin of the British Psychological Society* **5**: 13–19.

Garton A, Pratt P (1989). *Learning to be Literate: The Development of Spoken and Written Language*, Oxford: Basil Blackwell.

Gillingham A, Stillman BW (1969). *Remedial Training for Children with Specific Disability in Reading, Writing, and Penmanship*, 5th edn. Cambridge, MA: Educational Publishing Co.

Goodman K, Burke CL (1972). *Reading Miscue Inventory Manual*, London: Collier Macmillan.

Gorrie B, Parkinson E (1995). *Phonological Awareness Procedure*, Northumberland: STASS Publications.

Goswami U (1986). Children's use of analogy in learning to read: a developmental study. *Journal of Experimental Child Psychology* **42**: 73–83.

Goswami U (1994). Reading by analogy. In: Hulme C, Snowling M (Eds), *Reading Development and Dyslexia*, London: Whurr Publishers Ltd.

Goswami U, Bryant P (1990). *Phonological Skills and Learning to Read*, Hove: Lawrence Erlbaum Associates Ltd.

Hagley F (1987). *Suffolk Sentence Reading Test*, Windsor: NFER Nelson.

Hatcher PJ (1994). *Sound Linkage: an Integrated Programme for Overcoming Reading Difficulties*, London: Whurr Publishers Ltd.

Hawker GT (1962). *Spell it Yourself*, Oxford: Oxford University Press.

Hickey K (1977). *Language Training Scheme*. Bath: Better Books.

Hickey K (1992). *Dyslexia: a Language Training Course for Teachers and Learners*. Available from the Dyslexia Institute, Staines.

Hinshelwood J (1917). *Congenital Word Blindness*, London: H.K.Lewis.

Holdaway D (1979). *The Foundations of Literacy*, Gosford, NSW: Ashton Scholastic.

Hooper JB (1972). The syllable in phonological theory. *Language* **48**: 525–540.

Hornsby B, Shear F (1975). *Alpha to Omega*, Oxford: Heinemann Educational.

Hulme C, Snowling M (1992). Deficits in output phonology: a cause of reading failure? *Cognitive Neuropsychology* **9**: 47–72.

Hulme C, Snowling M (Eds) (1994). *Reading Development and Dyslexia*, London: Whurr Publishers Ltd.

Hunt R (Compiler) ( ). *Fuzzbuzz Reading Books*, Oxford: Oxford University Press.

Hunt R (Compiler) ( ). *Oxford Reading Tree*, Oxford: Oxford University Press.

Johnson P (1990). *A Book of One's Own*. London: Hodder and Stoughton.

Just MA, Carpenter PA (1987). *The Psychology of Reading and Language Comprehension*, Boston, MA: Allyn and Bacon.

Lahey M (1988). *Language Disorders and Language Development*, New York: Macmillan.

Lees J, Urwin S (1991). *Children With Language Disorders*, London: Whurr Publishers Ltd.

Liberman IY, Shankweiler D, Fischer FW, Carter B (1974). Explicit syllable and phoneme segmentation in the young child. *Journal of Experimental Child Psychology* **18**: 201–212.

MacKay D, Thompson B, Shaub P (1978). *Breakthrough to Literacy*, London: Longman.

Maclean M, Bryant P, Bradley L (1987). Rhymes, nursery rhymes and reading in early childhood. *Merrill–Palmer Quarterly* **33**: 255–281.

Makaton National Curriculum Series. Part 1: Symbols. (1993). Margaret Walker (Ed.), Pub. The Makaton Vocabulary Project 1993, 31 Firwood Drive, Camberley, Surrey, UK.

Martin T (1989). *The Strugglers*, Milton Keynes: Open University Press.

Maxwell SE, Wallach GP (1984). The language-learning disabilities connection: symptoms of early language disability change over time. In: Wallach GP, Butler KG (Eds), *Language Learning Disabilities in School Age Children*, London: Williams and Wilkins.

McDougall S, Hulme C (1994). Short-term memory, speech rate and phonological awareness as predictors of learning to read. In: Hulme C, Snowling M (Eds), *Reading Development and Dyslexia*, London: Whurr Publishers Ltd.

Miles E (1992). *The Bangor Dyslexia Teaching System*, Whurr Publishers: London.

Miles M, Clifford V (1994). A way with words. *Special Children* **77** (September).

Miles TR, Miles E (1990). *Dyslexia: a Hundred Years On*, Milton Keynes: Open University Press.

Moon C (1990). Miscues made simple. *Child Education*, November: 42–43.

Mosely D, Nicol C (1986). *The A.C.E. Spelling Dictionary*, Learning Development Aids.

Muter V (1994). The influence of phonological awareness and letter knowledge on beginning reading and spelling development. In: Hulme C, Snowling M (Eds), *Reading Development and Dyslexia*, London: Whurr Publishers Ltd.

Nolan J (1976). *King of the Road*, Essex: Oliver and Boyd.

Orton ST (1925). Word-blindness in school children. *Archives of Neurology and Psychiatry* **14**: 581–615.

Orton ST (1937). *Reading, Writing and Speech Problems in Children*, London: Chapman & Hall.

Passey J (1993). *Cued Articulation*, Northumberland, UK: STASS Publications.

Patterson KE, Coltheart V (1987). Phonological processes in reading: a tutorial review. In: Coltheart M (Ed.), *Attention and Performance XII: The Psychology of Reading*, pp. 421–448. London: Lawrence Erlbaum Associates.

Peters ML, Smith B (1993). *Spelling in Context: Strategies for Teachers and Learners*, Windsor: NFER Nelson.

Pinker S (1994). *The Language Instinct; The New Science of Language and Mind*, London: Penguin Press.

Rack JP, Snowling MJ, Olson RK (1992). The nonword reading deficit in developmental dyslexia: A review. *Reading Research Quarterly* **27/1**: 29–53.

Rayner K, Pollatsek A (1987). Eye movements in reading: a tutorial review. In: Coltheart M (Ed.). *Attention and Performance 11: The Psychology of Reading*, pp. 327–362. London: Lawrence Erlbaum Associates.

Read C (1971). Pre-school children's knowledge of English phonology: *Harvard Educational Review* **41**: 1–34.

Read C (1986). *Children's Creative Spelling*, London: Routledge and Kegan Paul.

Rosen M (1990). *The Hypnotiser*, London: Harper Collins.

Schonell FJ (1950). *Diagnostic and Attainment Testing*, Edinburgh: Oliver and Boyd.

Sinclair J (ed.) (1991). *Word Formation*, Collins Cobuild English Guide, London: Harper Collins.

Singleton C (1994). *Computers and Dyslexia: Educational Applications of New Technology*, Hull: BDA Computer Resource Centre.

Snowling M (1987). *Dyslexia: A Cognitive Developmental Perspective*, Oxford: Basil Blackwell.

Snowling M, Thomson ME (Eds) (1991) *Dyslexia. Integrating Theory and Practice*, London: Whurr Publishers Ltd.

Snowling MJ, Stothard S, McLean J (1996). *Graded Nonword Reading Test*, Suffolk, UK: Thames Valley Test Co.

SRA Corrective Reading (Decoding and Comprehension) (1988). Science Research Associates Ltd, Newtown Road, Henley-on-Thames, Oxfordshire, UK.

Stackhouse J (1989). Relationship between spoken and written language disorders . In: Mogford K, Sadler J (Eds). *Child Language Disability; Implications in an Educational Setting*, Cleveden, Philadelphia and Adelaide: Multilingual Matters Ltd.

Stackhouse J (1990). *Phonological Deficits in Developmental Reading and Spelling Disorders*, Edinburgh: Churchill Livingstone.

Stackhouse J, Wells B (1992). Dyslexia: the obvious and hidden speech and language disorder. In: Snowling M, Thomson ME (Eds), *Dyslexia: Integrating Theory and Practice*, London: Whurr Publishing Ltd.

Stone C, Franks E, Nicholson M (1992). *Beat Dyslexia!* LDA, Duke Street, Wisbech, Cambs. PE13 2AE.

Sunshine Books, Oxford: Heinemann Educational.

Thomson ME (1984). *Developmental Dyslexia; Its Nature, Assessment and Remediation*, London: Edward Arnold.

Thomson ME, Watkins EJ (1990). *Dyslexia. A Teaching Handbook*, London: Whurr Publishers Ltd.

Treiman R (1992). The role of intrasyllabic units in learning to read and spell. In: Gough PB, Ehri LC, Treiman R (Eds), *Reading Acquisition*, New Jersey: Laurence Erlbaum Associates.

Treiman R, Baron J (1981). Segmental analysis: development and relation to reading ability. In: MacKinnon GC, Waller TG (Eds), *Reading Research: Advances in Theory and Practice*, Vol. 3. New York: Academic Press.

Treiman R, Zukowski A (1991). Levels of phonological awareness. In: Brady SA, Shankweiler DP (Eds), *Phonological Processes in Literacy: A Tribute to Isabelle Y. Liberman*, pp 67–83. Hillsdale, NJ: Lawrence Erlbaum Associates.

Tunmer WE, Bower JA (1984). Metalinguistic awareness and reading acquisition. In: Tunmer WE, Pratt C, Herriman ML (Eds), *Metalinguistic Awareness in Children: Theory, Research and Implications*, Berlin: Springer–Verlag.

Van Kleek MA (1984). Metalinguistic skills: cutting across spoken and written language and problem solving abilities. In: Wallach G, Butler K (Eds), *Language Learning Disabilities in School-age Children*, London: Williams and Wilkins.

Van Oosteroom J, Devereux K (1992). *The Rebus Glossary*, LDA, Duke Street, Wisbech, Cambs, UK (first published as *Learning with Rebuses Glossary*, by EARO 1985).

Vygotsky LS (1978). *Mind in Society: The Development of Higher Psychological Processes*, Cambridge, Mass: Harvard University Press.

Wells G (1986). *The Meaning Makers: Children Learning to Use Language and Using Language to Learn*, London: Hodder and Stoughton.

Wheldall K, Merrett F, Colmar S (1987). Effective tutoring of low progress readers; pause, prompt and praise. *Support for Learning 2/1* (February): 5–12.

Whitehead MR (1990). *Language and Literacy in the Early Years*, London: Paul Chapman Publishing.

Index

Of related interest:

THIS BOOK DOESN'T MAKE ~~SENS~~ ~~CENS~~ ~~SNS~~ ~~SCENS~~ SENSE
Jean Augur
1995   ISBN 1 897635 13 3   paperback   reissue

THE HICKEY MULTISENSORY LANGUAGE COURSE
Edited by Jean Augur and Suzanne Briggs
1992   ISBN 1 870332 52 0   paperback   2 ed

MATHEMATICS FOR DYSLEXICS: A TEACHING HANDBOOK
S.J. Chinn and J.R. Ashcroft
1993   ISBN 1 870332 74 1   paperback

TACKLING DYSLEXIA: THE BANGOR WAY
Ann Cooke
1992   ISBN 1 870332 14 8   paperback

DYSLEXIA: AN INTRODUCTORY GUIDE
James Doyle
1995   ISBN 1 897635 67 2   paperback

DYSLEXIA MATTERS
Edited by Gerald Hales
1994   ISBN 1 897635 11 7   paperback

SOUND LINKAGE: AN INTEGRATED PROGRAMME FOR
OVERCOMING READING DIFFICULTIES
Peter Hatcher
1994   ISBN 1 897635 31 1

DYSLEXIA: PARENTS IN NEED
Pat Heaton
1996   ISBN 1 897635 73 7   paperback

DEALING WITH DYSLEXIA
Pat Heaton and Patrick Winterson
1996   ISBN 1 897635 57 5   paperback

READING DEVELOPMENT AND DYSLEXIA
Edited by Charles Hulme and Margaret Snowling

1994 ISBN 1 897635 85 0 paperback
ADULT DYSLEXIA: ASSESSMENT, COUNSELLING AND TRAINING
David McLoughlin, Gary Fitzgibbon and Vivienne Young
1993 ISBN 1 897635 35 4 paperback

THE BANGOR DYSLEXIA TEACHING SYSTEM
Elaine Miles
1992 ISBN 1 870332 59 8 paperback 2 ed

DYSLEXIA: THE PATTERN OF DIFFICULTIES
T.R. Miles
1993 ISBN 1 870332 39 3 paperback 2 ed

DYSLEXIA AND STRESS
Edited by T.R. Miles and V. Varma
1995 ISBN 1 897635 22 2 paperback

INSTRUMENTAL MUSIC FOR DYSLEXICS
Sheila Oglethorpe
1996 ISBN 1 897635 69 9 paperback

DYSLEXIA, SPEECH AND LANGUAGE: A PRACTITIONER'S
HANDBOOK
Edited by Margaret Snowling and Joy Stackhouse
1996 ISBN 1 897635 48 6 paperback

DYSLEXIA: INTEGRATING THEORY AND PRACTICE
Edited by Margaret Snowling and Michael E. Thomson
1991 ISBN 1 870332 47 4 paperback

DEVELOPMENTAL DYSLEXIA
Michael E. Thomson
1989 ISBN 1 870332 70 9 paperback 3 ed

DYSLEXIA: A TEACHING HANDBOOK
Michael E. Thomson and Bill Watkins
1990 ISBN 1 870332 06 7 paperback

Whurr Publishers' complete catalogue is available upon request.